Ivor Felstein

Sex and the
Longer Life

Allen Lane
The Penguin Press

For Lawrence Hatton

S B N 7139 0142 X

Printed in Great Britain by
Lowe & Brydone (Printers) Ltd, London
Set in Linotype Times

Contents

Contents

Introduction

One of the pleasant aspects of specializing in a relatively new branch of medicine is that people are always asking me to give talks or lectures on my special subject. My pleasure derives not from the free cups of tea which ladies' guilds proffer so liberally but from the opportunity to address a captive audience and explain just what modern medicine is trying to achieve in the older age groups of the community. In other words, I am an unashamed propagandist for the work which is being done in geriatrics today and I welcome every opportunity to enlighten individuals and groups on this work. At question time following a talk, a recurring theme of many occasions is the inquiry 'what is the point of doctors keeping us alive so much longer, if a longer life means poor health, low income, and lack of youthful pleasures?' Health, or lack of it, is progressively important to all of us as we grow older and is a preoccupation of all social classes and both sexes. It is a vested interest of rich and poor, and is a driving force for both the preventive and therapeutic branches of the National Health Service. Low income, that is the fixed income of retirement or pension with or without the falling value of monies from other sources such as savings or annuities, is another preoccupation of later years for a substantial section of the community. It affects the way of life, the domestic comforts and the individual nutrition of older people, and is a driving force for government departments like the Ministry of

Introduction

Social Security* and for local authority departments like the Welfare and Social Services.

'Lack of youthful pleasures' is a rather vague sort of phrase which might cover anything from being unable to enjoy a fast game of soccer or tennis, to being unable to eat a vast variety of foods, or to being unable to enjoy the freedom of social interchange and non-conformity in dress and speech of the current generation of youth. It may also be taken to imply the likely absence of sexual pleasure, if not of sex itself, in later life. Or again it may be a phrase which is used simply to remind us nostalgically of a happy irrecoverable past, of days when we combined ambition with no thought of failure and zest in living with no thought of dying. Direct questions on sex in later life rarely arise following my talks. This may be due to the 'spiritual' environment of the church hall precluding earthly inquiries. It may be due to the absence of any interest or thoughts on sex in later life, or, alternatively, to shyness and modesty at airing ideas and views in open discussion. Since the odd question that does arise – I mean occasional but they are sometimes odd – is often concerned with abnormal sexual behaviour in an older relative or friend, it may be that a doctor is viewed as being interested in sick behaviour only. This is not true and in fact he is just as interested in healthy behaviour, both from the point of view of preventive medical therapy and for the reason of obtaining a yardstick by which to judge sick behaviour.

The idea of writing a manuscript on sex in the longer life of twentieth-century man and woman had occurred to me some years ago. There were several pointers as to its possible value. In the first instance, I felt it might help to dispel some of the fog which surrounds sexual behaviour in our society. Many sexologists have issued into print on sexual morality and *mores* in the young single and young married

*Now the Department of Health and Social Security.

8

community groups but few have braved the middle-age groups and less than a handful have considered the sexual needs and activities of men and women in the over-fifty category. Secondly, I felt that a monograph on sex in the longer life would help to balance the picture of life in later years, which seems to be framed as a period of low tensions and low output, on a background of diminishing physical health and poor mental energy. Thirdly, I considered that sexual activity in older people has a rightful place in the sociology of the modern community and a manuscript which revealed and interpreted this activity should add to the improved understanding of health and illness in older age groups of all social classes.

When I chatted to a number of people about the value of such a book being written, I was greeted as might be expected with a wide range of reactions. These varied from the facetious: 'You're just trying to cheer yourself up for your own old age', to the anxious: 'I'd certainly like to know more about the dangers of sex when you're old', to the gloomy: 'What's the point of writing about a sex life that isn't', to the supercilious 'Is the time ripe to tell ordinary people about sex in later life?' Such responses were governed by both the personal attitude to sex in general and the professional outlook on sexual problems in particular. The two outstanding comments which finally determined my writing this manuscript were given to me by the same person. One moment he said, 'You would be better researching and writing about the causes of tissue cancer in older people.' The next moment he queried, 'Do older people really have a sex life?'

In a Western community which, as ours does, lays great stress on the fullness of adolescent and young adult life, the last question of the preceding paragraph should not come as a surprise. Young people readily equate ageing with a decline in sexual potency. This loss of sexual power is

Introduction

further linked in the young mind with an absence of sexual desire and a loss of sexual interest in older people. Since, in any case, older people rarely broadcast the continued healthy function of their sexual organs, the young person's equation of older years with absence of sex is not consciously denied. Moreover older parents do not overtly confirm their enjoyment of continued sexual relations to their children even if the latter are 'young marrieds'. The loss of the marriage partner through death or divorce, or the absence of a marriage partner through intended or unintended celibacy, acts as a further inhibiting influence on the oral or written expression of older peoples' sexual urges and needs. Popular expressions confirm the attitude that youth and strong sexual urge go together: 'he's a lad with a roving eye', while age and absence of sexual urge usually go together: 'he's well past it'. As a logical extension of such an attitude, the old man with a roving eye is denigrated as a 'dirty old man'.

This view of absent sexual interest and lack of sexual desire of older people may be prevalent not only in young and poorly informed members of the community but also in somewhat older and scientific members such as doctors, psychologists and sociologists. Both in day-to-day consideration and in long-term planning these influential people may give low priority to sexual activity in older people when appraising the social and economic needs and physical and mental health problems of a longer life. This is more likely where these scientists, otherwise enlightened in their own specialities, adopt the favoured attitudes of the secular and religious establishments towards sex. However, such professional people are called upon by the community to give advice on sexual as well as other problems. They may be asked to comment critically on contemporary *mores*. They may be invited to guide parental or authority attitudes in families and groups respectively. For that reason, they must examine the facts and the evidence and keep abreast of changing ideas and new knowledge of sexual function in later life. Some of this information comes from previous and current social and medical studies in the major Western communities including our own and those of the Americas. Further evidence in this country is likely from questionnaire studies and factual surveys in preventive and screening clinics, health centres and private group studies. Personal discussions and careful study of the available literature and meetings with relatives, other doctors, health workers, social and research workers have all helped me to set out the views and conclusions reached in this book.

Such views and conclusions may, it is hoped, be used validly for personal encouragement and for the purpose of sex counselling. For there is no doubt that we are living in an era in which sex counselling has become a primary sociological interest. A glance at women's journals or at magazines and digests or at Sunday and weekday newspapers reveals the recurring theme of sexual advice. This advice is directed towards the adolescent and the young single and married people in the main but also towards middle-aged people at times. The information may be presented in didactic essay form, in thematic letters to the editor, in question and answer columns, as part of a friendly columnist's weekly ritual, or as sensational or exposé material.

The reasons for the popularity of the written, rather than the oral, form of sex counselling stem from the 'third party' anonymity of the questioner in relation to the columnist. Outsiders to the world of the 'problem pages' are inclined to treat the sex questions as a huge joke. They scorn the naïvety of the questioner and scoff at the seriousness of the reply.

The columnists themselves know, however, that for every frivolous letter there may be a hundred letters with genuine sexual problems and that, unfortunately, these are often not easily resolved by simple advice in print or under plain cover.

There are certain groups of active 'social workers' in the community who are well aware of the sex problems in marriage and within families. Not only family doctors but also midwives, health visitors, almoners and child guidance workers, for example, recognize the sexual vulnerability of such population groups as adolescents, newly-weds, first child couples and menopausal couples. Directly or indirectly, these 'social workers' may be called upon to play the role of sex counsellor to individuals or families. This role may be charged to them as figures of authority – as are also ministers of religion and schoolteachers – or as professionals in medicine or nursing, or as friends of the family, or simply as people who are good listeners. These 'social workers', especially if they are older or more mature than those who seek advice from them, are presumed to have had sexual experience, and their attitude and under-standing of sex to have profited by that experience. This may or may not be the case in fact. Certainly it is clear that some individuals are more able to grasp the essentials of a sexual problem, whatever their professional training or standing, and to apply this imaginatively and pragmatic-ally to the situation for the best solution. Of course, advice on sex may be given gratuitously where a 'social worker' thinks the situation calls for it, as well as being directly requested. Like all forms of advice – and I recognize this fact for this book – it may be subsequently ignored, acted upon or used to manipulate people or situations for private or public ends.

Some people welcome the role of sex counsellor. This welcome may be based on a genuine interest in the welfare of others or as an opportunity to propagate their personal viewpoint. Either way, people are often ready to give advice on sex which is based on their own limited experience or on hearsay evidence or on the basis of 'sound commonsense'. For example, a midwife would recognize that a mother of one child who offered another mother 'in labour' advice on delivering the child, was clearly unqualified to do so and might give dangerous advice accordingly. The same midwife might nevertheless counsel a mother on a sex problem and the counsel be based only on the experience of her own married life. Such counsel may be reasonable or even valid in the circumstances. Yet as a scientifically trained person she will know the importance of statistical analysis of group experience, and advice based on a wider knowledge of the facts. This rational approach may be forgotten only because it is a sexual problem.

While sex itself can be regarded as instinctive, based on hormonal physiology, the sexual tensions and sexual needs of individuals contain as large a psychic element as a physical one. The development of the sexual psyche is complex and includes parental influence and family upbringing. Within the family unit, it is the emotional bond between the growing infant and child and his or her mother and father that is significant. Mutual affection and love as well as parental acceptance affect the sexual psyche in a positive maturation of thought and behaviour. At a later phase, the psyche develops further when its erotic content is directed towards a member of the opposite or the same sex in the real world outside the family unit. Here again, acceptance and mutual affection establish sexual confidence and augment sexual maturation: or rejection promotes sexual inferiority and encourages sexual inadequacy, as the case may be. Both fictional and factual literature abound with examples of how the first 'falling in love' profoundly affects the sexual progress of the individual. To these influences must be added the basic intelligence quotient and subsequent educational level as well as the original and subsequent social class of the particular person. Within the social class, the sexual psyche is further affected by the ethnic and cultural background and onto this is grafted the religious training of the individual. Yet another factor is the influence of the occupation which the person follows, particularly in the early post-school or post-university years. This complex development is true for both the counsellor and the counselled, and both sides must be aware how this growth of their sexual psyche will influence the attitude to the problem as well as the advice likely to be given. Unfortunately this awareness may only be a superficial sort as few of us have the time or the opportunity or the economic means to undergo psychoanalysis for a deeper understanding.

I have mentioned above that some people feel that sex counselling can be adequately undertaken on the basis of 'sound commonsense'. In this book I have tried to avoid the type of commonsense which is based on the logic of a single immediate experience. The extrapolation of such logic is unreliable and may be downright unhelpful. However I have admitted the use of commonsense where the general facts and group knowledge make its use for advice technically sound and more cogent.

It is an interesting coincidence that at the time I was preparing a final revision of this book there was a resurgence of interest in the 'youth pill' and the 'youth injection' therapy practised on the other side of the Iron Curtain. Based on the use of procaine introduced by the Bucharest doctor Anna Aslan, the therapy is alleged to postpone the ageing process and tone up the whole body. It is further alleged that this therapy increases sexual vigour and improves the memory. Thankfully it does not claim to make one young again but merely to 'postpone the ageing process'.

It does not seem ten years since Professor Aslan visited

Great Britain to talk to medical audiences about her work with procaine in the older age groups. Official medical opinion in this country then, as now, was strongly sceptical of her claims for rejuvenation of patients by procaine alone. Some doctors thought that mild physiological effects might result from an effect of procaine on the adrenal glands. Others felt that most of the success apparently achieved by the injections was the combined result of 'needling' and hypno-suggestion. With regard to renewal of sexual vigour, the importance of psychic support is stressed in Chapter Four and no doubt the psychic support of the Aslan procaine patients has contributed to the alleged successes, particularly in the sex function aspects, in older patients. Whatever the truth about the 'youth pill', the recurring interest in the prolongation of sexual powers and the potentiation of sexual function in older people is clearly manifested on a universal scale. It is hoped sincerely that this book may amplify such interest and increase the sexual perspective.

1 | The Changing Climate

The New Old Age

A hundred years ago, when the poet Tennyson wrote his celebrated poem on the death of King Arthur of the Round Table, old age was viewed as the fourth decade of life. As the legendary king moved to his end, 'the old order yielding place to new', the writer of 'Idylls of the King' did not foresee a time when life would begin with renewed vigour at forty instead of ending there. The truth of a longer life and a later old age is more than just a happy piece of advertising copy for vitamin or phosphate merchandisers to cast in our direction. In 1868 the expectation of life for the newborn baby was forty years. As I write in 1968, the life expectation for today's infant is a remarkable seventy years. Moreover, for those already reaching the age of forty, there is a further expectation of life for another twenty years. Many factors have contributed to this improvement in life span over a period of a hundred years. Some of these are well-known and others are less familiar.

The first major progress point was the development of public health measures in the towns and cities of Great Britain. The introduction of sewage collection and disposal and the application of animal and human quarantine programmes was forced upon a population repeatedly savaged by outbreaks of epidemic disease. The initial reluctance was soon overcome when the success of the measures began to eliminate the killer infectious diseases. Two more public health plans, namely food hygiene control and mass vaccination, really brought the control and virtual elimination of typhoid and diphtheria, as well as plague, rabies, cholera and typhus.

The next point of progress was the discovery of the vitamins. These essential food factors were found to be missing in certain widespread and disabling diseases. Two vitamin deficiency illnesses which afflicted the community were scurvy and rickets. These were controlled and virtually eliminated with the discoveries of vitamins C and D respectively.

Almost in parallel with better understanding of nutritional illnesses came the developments in maternity and child care. Better understanding of illness in pregnancy and the introduction of anaesthesia and operative procedures for delivery reduced both the maternal death toll and the risk to the unborn child. Improved care of premature infants and improved knowledge of nourishing infants and children lowered the death and morbidity rate of the under-fives.

For adults especially, the next point of progress was the discovery that certain previously fatal illnesses could be controlled and death averted by replacement therapy. For example, sugar diabetes could be controlled by injecting insulin that the affected patient's body was no longer producing. Also, for example, pernicious anaemia could be corrected and controlled by lifelong replacement injections of cyanocobalamin.

Apart from the progressive improvements in all branches of surgical treatment and in anaesthetics, the last really major breakthrough was the discovery of chemotherapy. In this, the development of sulphonamides, penicillin and streptomycin spelt the end for the flourishing bacterial illnesses such as lobar pneumonia, tuberculosis and streptococcal fevers. The antibiotic era, as it is called, has cleared the way for doctors to tackle the remaining three great killers, namely cancer, virus disease and the degenerative illnesses such as coronary thrombosis and strokes.

If we consider the background outlined above, the major reason for a longer life is clearer. It is mainly due to the elimination and control of diseases and deficiencies at the childhood and young adult end of life, rather than being due to the improvement of health in the over-sixty age groups. This is a result both of the public health needs that initiated progress and of the concentration of medical research in the past five decades. Even after the arrival of the National Health Service in this country in 1948, government-sponsored and privately sponsored laboratory and clinical investigation work has focused on the young life, as if the old life was not worth considering. The first inroad into this traditional concentration on youth began with the gerontologist and progressed with the geriatrician. The former began to study the processes of ageing, both animal and human, and the mechanisms responsible or possibly causal in ageing. They also use the scientific method of gerontology to assess behaviour in the ageing animal or human.

As a corollary to gerontology, physicians interested in the diagnosis and treatment of diseases in older people developed the medical speciality of geriatrics. This speciality uses not only the knowledge derived from gerontology but also the general medical understanding of illness and disability in the human body.

The great stimulus to geriatrics appeared in 1948 when Dr J. H. Shedon published his now famous monograph 'The Social Medicine of Old Age'. Doctors and social workers alike were startled at the findings of this report on how old people lived, what illnesses and disabilities they suffered and what was needed to help them improve their lot. The Medical Society for the Care of the Elderly (afterwards the British Geriatrics Society) was founded the same year as Sheldon published his work. This society, in particular, encouraged the growth of hospital geriatric units for the diagnosis and treatment of disability and illness in later life. Social work departments and welfare departments of local health authorities undertook their own surveys of the needs and problems of older members of the community. On the basis of their findings, community care projects have been introduced. These include, for example, the home helps service. Voluntary bodies have also taken an interest in social and remedial work for older people and support such services as meals-on-wheels and citizens' advice bureaux.

Psychologists have also been studying the effects of ageing on personality and mental state. They have considered changes in skill and aptitude as well as alterations in behaviour or actual mental disorder. Their work has shown the strategies and art of adjustment in successful adaptation to the later years of the longer life. It has also revealed many of the problems arising from unsuccessful adaptation.

This new interest and new understanding of older people's physical and mental state has improved the outlook for the new old age of the second half of the twentieth century – the years from sixty to ninety. A major omission in the study and understanding of our new old age, however, concerns the sexual behaviour and sexual needs of middle-aged and older people. If you read the social and cultural studies of groups of old people which have been published in this country, there is never, or rarely, a line on the sex function in these groups. Books or monographs on the biological aspects of ageing stress the deterioration of the sexual organs, often in such a way as to confirm the idea that there can be no sex life in later years. Psychological studies are often more interested in abnormal sexual behaviour in later years than in normal sex functions and needs. The family doctor or specialist to whom the older person may turn for advice on sexual matters may himself have difficulty in handling sexual problems or guiding his older patients' sexual activities because of lack of medical data and lack of medical training in this aspect of social life.

Many professional people on this side of the Atlantic who have been initially interested in the investigation and propagation of the facts of sexual life in any age group, have been discouraged by the reaction of establishment groups. They find it hard to persuade the leaders of suitable authorities to undertake group investigation on a medical or medical-social basis. Some progress has been made with the younger age groups but the source stimulus has been from the criminal or disturbed behaviour problems of teenage and young adult communities. Little has been forthcoming from the adjusted and lawful section of the community. My own efforts to obtain a research grant some years ago confirm the apathy towards obtaining the facts. I applied to a large industrial concern with a major interest in birth control for research funds to study group data on sexual function in certain older age groups in England. After a sympathetic correspondence, my application for a research grant was turned down. Neither did the industrial concern offer reconsideration for a future year. The impression I received was that 'this kind of work is really not important'.

When studies are undertaken, however, the findings suggest that in older age groups sexual function is not inconsiderable and should not readily be brushed aside as unimportant. A famous retrospective study of centenarians highlights this point. That particular study revealed that in their younger years this group had stable marriages which the partners (and the researcher) regarded as mentally and physically satisfactory. Moreover there were more children per couple than the national average. Further, where one spouse died, the remarriage rate was again higher than the average and this was true even in the eighth and ninth decades. In the same study, it was noted that sexual activity in the group was little affected by the loss of reproductive capacity in either or both partners. Admittedly, people who have reached a hundred years of age in the middle of the twentieth century are a special group. They have survived natural and man-made disasters as well as major and epidemic diseases, not to mention nine decades of stress. Still, distinctive as these centenarians are even among the older members of the community, they are an important example of the fact that sexual interest and function do continue in later years.

We have noted already how the general expectation of life at birth has improved considerably in the last hundred years. As yet, however, there has been very little change in the expectation of life for the man or woman over sixty. Doctors are not too dismayed at this because, as we have also noted, certain illnesses in the over-sixties that were once fatal or disabling can now be cured or well controlled. This means that the longer life and its later years can be made healthier and more vigorous for the individual. Work and leisure can be enjoyed better and society can continue to benefit from the experience and skills of its older members. Better health in later life can and should include better maintenance of sexual function for both sexes. It should also ensure that sexual satisfaction and fulfilment can continue well into old age and be a recognized social function for this age group. Return to good health after illness at any age brings many joys and one of these is the resumption of sexual relations. As one of my older patients once told me: 'I'm not quite better, doctor, I'm not chasing the wife yet.'

Five Basic Ideas

We have remarked in the introduction to this book that our current Western society is much preoccupied with the fullness of adolescent and young adult life. Implicit in that fullness is the possession of much sexual energy and satisfactory sources for the release or employment of this energy. The strong link between sexual function and youthfulness has been forged by a number of basic ideas, of which there are at least five important ones I should like to consider in this chapter. The first idea is that sexual function is purely for procreation. On this basis, the young are likely to be the most fertile. The second idea is that sexual tension is built mainly on physical attraction between the sexes, and that maintenance of this tension is fortified by physical attractiveness. On this basis, boys and girls with the 'bloom of youth' should have the greatest and most prolonged sexual tension. The third idea is that sexual tension and the need for outlet are always highest in youth and decline quickly towards middle age. On this basis, old people would have no sexual tension and no need for sexual outlet.

The fourth idea which links sex function and youth is the proposition that romantic love, with its imaginative delights and psycho-physical passion, can only occur in youth and young adulthood. The fifth idea for consideration is that, among other factors which make youth the choicest setting for sexual function, the body organs in young people are at peak health levels. On this basis, the longer life goes on, the less likely is it that the internal and external organs connected with sexual function will be at optimum levels. The overall effect would be that sex in later life is less satisfying physically and consequently less satisfying psychically as well.

These five basic ideas are not individually mutually exclusive. There is obviously, for example, a connexion between the physical attraction idea and the highest sexual tension in youth idea. For our purpose, however, we can here consider the ideas separately and see whether the premises stand or fall on the facts.

The first idea, then, links sexual function, procreation and youthful fertility. Lay people as well as physiologists and zoologists come to the obvious conclusion, from observation of the products of sexual activity in animals, that the teleological explanation of this activity is the continuation of the species. In the human being sexual function similarly ensures continuation of the human species.

Sexual activity in animals reveals both the instinctive urge and pleasurable gratification. In human beings both these elements are present also, and in addition humans have language in which to express what they feel. Words uttered by sexual partners before, during and after the sexual act confirm that the intercourse is an expression of love and happiness and not merely an act intended to beget children. Through his capacity for abstract thought and interpretative action the human being enlarges the basic premise for sex. Moreover, Freud has taught us that the energy of the human being's sexual urge and drive can be transferred in alternative directions. This sublimated libido is said to be the basis of creative endeavour in the artistic and literary and commercial fields, for example.

Even for those who consider sexual function is purely for procreation, that function need not be so emphatically linked with youth as tentatively suggested in the first basic idea quoted above. Now the capacity to conceive and reproduce varies between male and female. This variation lies in age of onset and age of regression. For the female from the start of ovulation at about the age of twelve to the end of menstruation in the late forties there are roughly four decades of possible conception. For the male, from the start of ejaculation of active semen at about thirteen or fourteen until the decline of active semen in the seventies, or even eighties, there may be roughly seven decades of possible fertilization of a female partner. These facts show us that procreation is not confined to youthful fertility but that fertility can be just as likely for the older man.

However, the opinion that sexual function is purely for procreation and that each sexual union should have conception in prime view is still present in the Western community today. It is embodied in the section of Christian religion which still holds strong to the teachings of St Augustine. Among the latter we find that sexual function in general is viewed warily and is tied up dangerously with sin. Marital intercourse is permitted, however, as part of the sacrament of marriage provided each act may naturally end in conception. (This does not necessarily exclude sexual intercourse for infertile couples or post-menopausal women, a point considered again on page 140). Birth control by mechanical interference is consequently viewed as sinful. This includes 'the pill', a view which has again been ratified by the Papacy at the time of writing.

Fortunately, however, the current view which prevails is a secular one and not the somewhat ascetic religious one. That is, the sexual function is seen as an important psychophysical expression, mutually necessary to man and woman. In the marriage setting, it is seen as a stabilizing influence in marital adjustment and a factor in the maturing of the conjugal relationship. Within this setting the sexual act may be a source of happiness and pleasure as well as the chosen moment for conception of wanted children. This secular view puts, as it were, children in their place. It also leads us to see that sexual function in people who are no longer fertile by virtue of their age in years can still be important and meaningful. (As a corollary, it also means young people who are infertile for organic reasons can still enjoy their sexual function. There, the family unit may be completed by the adoption or fostering of children.)

Returning to our first idea I have suggested that 'the young are likely to be *most* fertile'. Certainly the maximum frequency of sexual outlet is highest in adolescence and the twenties in men. Assuming the outlet is sexual intercourse in the married group of this age – and assuming the health of the semen – the chances of fertilization are greater than in the older age group by virtue of this frequency. In women the highest frequency of sexual intercourse occurs in the late twenties and the frequency stays at a high level into the early forties. This encourages the possibility of pregnancy in a group which can no longer be classified under the heading of youth. Illness affecting the sexual organs and hence the ability to bear children, can occur at any age in the otherwise fertile years. The venereal diseases are more likely to affect the fertility of younger age groups, while the degenerative illnesses, like hardening of the arteries, affect older age groups. Other facts which affect the fertility rate include contraception of any kind for social or medical reasons, and psychological disturbances of a minor or major nature. Deficiencies of sex hormones or pituitary hormones may also play a part. Thus, if I rephrase the idea as 'the young are likely to be more fertile but that fertility persists into middle age for women and old age for men', the link idea of youth, procreation and sexual function is considerably weakened.

The second idea is that sexual tension is built mainly on physical attraction between the sexes. From this it is inferred that the more attractive the physical appearance the greater the chances of sexual attachment and the better the outlook for the fulfilment of sexual function. Girls and boys with the 'bloom of youth' are consequently likely to have these greater chances, and older people who have lost this bloom would have relatively fewer chances. The relationship between attractive physical appearance and sexual attractiveness is far from being clear cut. Certainly a handsome boy or a beautiful girl will be noticed by the opposite sex and may be praised or admired for that handsomeness or beauty. It does not necessarily mean that every admirer will also appraise that handsomeness or beauty in sexual terms and be sexually aroused and sexually attracted.

Both for men and women, the advertising industry for commerce strongly encourages the idea of a relationship between good looks and sex. Not only foundation garments, cosmetics and overclothes are 'sold' to us on this basis but books (by their dustjackets) and records (by their outer sleeves). The good looks and sex theme is further intensified in the glamour that surrounds such industries as films, television and the stage, not to mention modelling and professional beauty competitions. It says much for the practicality of human beings, however, that despite this constant harangue which insists that products should be bought for their potential sex value, we buy but are not really sold. People dress up and apply cosmetics for their own pleasure and the admiration of their own sex as well as for the opposite sex. They are both conforming to certain social standards and complementing an external visual image. Thus even the wedding-day couple, whose sexual attraction to each other may be taken for granted, combine social conformity with a visual image of physical attractiveness in white bridal gown and grey morning suit respectively. To the onlookers they make a handsome couple as they walk down the aisle, a thought which subconsciously extends to the bed chamber.

The physical pairing of couples, then, is more than just a simple function of attractive physical appearance. Look around you in the dance hall or cinema, in the bowling alley or concert hall, at the card evening or variety club and see at a glance the heterogenous physical appearances of couples. There is no clearly defined mating of physical types so that partner attraction must be more subtle and more complex than good 'vital statistics' or handsome physique. In fact mutual attraction arises through frequency of meeting at work or in leisure places, and through expressions of understanding of problems and ambitions, and through participation in cultural or educational interests, for example. The drawing together may be slow or quick, may be a function of time to spare or little time to waste, or even the result of an intentional arrangement by a third (matchmaking) party.

Once the physical attraction has begun or proceeded then a romantic overlay of 'falling in love' may well enhance the physical appearance of each of the partners as seen by the other. This romantically enhanced physical attractiveness certainly helps to maintain the sexual tension between the partners. Moreover, it helps to continue the theme as promulgated among the youth of today that attractive physical appearance means more chance and better maintenance of sexual tension. The playwright Paddy Chayevsky showed us very clearly in his play and film, *Marty*, the pernicious influence of the glamour and sex theme on the plain girl and the homely (American sense) boy. They are treated intolerably by the society which values good looks and extrovert personality and drawn together sympathetically in their mutual problem of being 'undesirables'. In an Eastern society, where the matchmaker or marriage go-between considered prospective pairings on personality, aptitudes, social skills, income and health, a client's attractive physical appearance was merely a bonus to possible pairing. In Western society where matchmaking is no longer fashionable although still discreetly practiced, physical appearance is given a higher rating.

In the face of this promotion of the glamour of youth, older people seen on films or television or in social or working groups find their external appearance regarded less wholesomely. Individual sections of their anatomy, from head to legs, are contrasted with those of their younger companions to the older person's detriment. The extension of this is to assume that older people, less pleasing in appearance, are less sexually attractive both to each other and to younger people. This again is not borne out by a consideration of the physical appearances of older partners who enjoy sexual relations within or outside the marital bond. As with younger people, physical attraction is compounded of a number of personality traits, time and place factors and mutual desires and goals. And for older people, too, the romantic overlay of falling in love also adds to physical attraction and helps to maintain the sexual tension following arousal.

So the second idea, like the first, has to be amended. It can be better phrased that 'physical attraction which helps maintain sexual tension does not necessarily infer beauty or good looks'. Further, youth has no prerogative in physical attraction which leads to sexual tension and attachment.

The third link idea which was proposed in the first paragraph of this chapter is that the need for sexual outlet is always highest in youth and declines quickly towards middle age. Extrapolating this to old age would lead us to conclude that old people have no sexual tension and no need for sexual outlet.

I have said before that the sexual urge may be regarded as instinctive, based on a given anatomical structure modified by physiological hormonal directives to nerves, muscles and blood vessels. On to this reflex of organs and tissues, the human being has grafted conditioning and technique and a complex mental aspect which alters the responses in a given individual. This mental modification of sexual response and patterns occurs in males and females and produces the wide varieties in sexual behaviour and outlet that form the spectrum of 'normal' sexual activity. What is sexually stimulating for one man may produce no reaction in another and a small reaction in a third. Moreover, if there is sexual arousal in the first man and little arousal in the third man, the second man in whom there is no reaction may consider the first man to have excessive sexual tension – oversexed in parlour parlance. The method of outlet for the first man may be erection with masturbation and for the third man a nocturnal wet dream while the second man has no need for outlet in the absence of arousal. Now whatever the second man may think, the three of them are within our 'normal' spectrum. For they are exhibiting responses (or lack of them) as a result of the sexual conditioning which has been developed through preferential experience.

The effects of preferential sexual experience can be expected to modify and variegate those objects or events which promote sexual tensions, at any age. Thus, if a boy has his first regular erections while watching a physically mature teenage girl running in the school races, he may be roused later by activities of the female partner which produce rise and fall in the breasts in the same rhythmic manner as racing. Further, he may find sexual tension simply in talking about this. Yet further, the effect is just as likely to occur at fifty as at twenty. The level of sexual tension is not so much a function of the individual male or female age, as of the provoking stimulus and the significance of that stimulus in terms of previous sexual experience. If the individual is mentally clear and his or her sexual apparatus is physically sound, then the sexual tension will rise to the level that is characteristic for that one individual. It is somewhat analogous to the psycho-physical aspects of pain sensation. For people who have a low pain threshold, i.e. a low tolerance to painful stimuli, a wasp sting may be experienced as a catastrophic and almost unbearable agony. For people with a progressively higher pain threshold the wasp sting becomes no more disastrous than the prick of an injection needle for a vaccination. But on to the tolerance of pain in physical terms is grafted the previous experience of pain-provoking situations and the responses of the time when they occurred.

It is reasonable to assume that any considerable rise in an individual's sexual tension will usually result in some form of sexual activity that acts as an outlet for this tension. Obviously the social circumstances in which the sexually roused individual finds himself or herself will influence the mode of outlet. Thus in an all-male setting such as a prison, masturbation or homosexual activity may be the outlet, while at an all-night New Year's Eve party intercourse may be the outlet, for male and for female.

Sexual tension can be provoked in a setting which our third-link idea would not lead us to expect. I remember a newly recruited lady craft-worker in her early twenties visiting a male long-stay ward in a geriatric unit of a northern hospital. A smiling coiffured blonde in a shift dress, she met each of the patients in the day area and those confined to bed, to try to interest them in such diversionary therapy as rug-making and basket-work. Some of these long-stay patients were normally apathetic and indifferent even to the passive entertainment of race meetings on television or free film presentations. The charge nurse complained to me in a good-natured way that most of the men required night sedation after the craft worker's visit. He was obviously perturbed that these normally 'well-behaved' old men had experienced sexual arousal at the visit of a pretty woman, a good example of the 'not at their age surely' reaction of younger people to sexual function in older people.

By contrast, I can recall the advice of a tutor physician when his male medical-student class visited the female wing of a tuberculosis sanatorium in the early 1950s. He warned the students that these ladies had been 'confined' to the hospital for anything from six to eighteen months so that the presence of active young men could produce a (sexually) inflammable atmosphere. Nobody thought that such a reaction might be 'bad behaviour' as with the old men's reaction above.

The original figures of Kinsey, Pomeroy and Nelson, and the work of Schofield some twenty years later, have shown us that, taking all forms of sexual activity and outlet into account, total sexual activity is highest from adolescence to the middle twenties. Once again, however, there is tremendous individual variation in frequency and type of outlet, again based on conditioning and socially modifying factors. These higher figures for younger people apply particularly to the males and include the premarital sexual activity of both sexes. The figures do show a slow but steady decline of total sexual outlet for both sexes over the years, but – and it is an important 'but' – there is no fixed end point for sexual activity at 'such and such an age'.

The third link idea, to return to our discussion, should be amended to read that 'sexual activity and outlet are highest in adolescence and youth but decline slowly over the years with no universally fixed end point'. It is not true that old people have no sexual tension and no need for sexual outlet.

In my own practice, which involves a wide range of middle-aged to older patients referred by family doctors, other specialists or preventive clinics, for example, my primary consideration is the diagnosis and treatment and return to health of the patients. Apart from their sickness, members of this heterogeneous group have little in common, since it covers both sexes, different social classes, different occupations (or former occupations) and different ethnic and religious groups. In the course of many case histories, from answers to discreet questions or from spontaneously given information, the presence of sexual tensions and the continuation of sexual outlet both in marriage and outside it has been clearly impressed on me. (Of course the good doctor is cautious about purely clinical impressions based on either the selective nature of the group he treats or his own pre-judged preferences and beliefs. This was one of the reasons why, as I explained in the earlier part of this chapter, I was so keen to initiate a statistically valid research project to confirm my clinical impression and that not only in patients but in recognizably well people too.)

The Spirit of Romance

We have seen in the last chapter how three of the basic ideas which link youth and sex and imply age and no sex, have to be modified in the light of current knowledge. The fourth and fifth link ideas are more difficult to assess because of the difficulties of defining romantic love on the one hand and health (as opposed to disease) on the other.

The fourth idea proposed that 'romantic love, with its imaginative delights and psycho-physical passion, can occur only in youth and young adulthood'. A picture of romantic love conjurs up an image of tender embraces, words of endearment, gifts for remembered anniversaries, sighing and heavy breathing in physical contact. Especially, however, the picture of romantic love evokes an image of intense pleasure, an 'out of this world' feeling, a blissful knowing that 'you are just right for each other', an ideal state of togetherness that transcends the mundane relationships of 'ordinary' people.

Looked at historically, it can be seen that the relationship between men and women in sexual terms has at times been dominantly practical and at times dominantly romantic. Before the emancipation of womanhood in suffrage, employment, and education, the paramount need for security as a wife and mother meant arranged or contrived marriages where romantic love was a rare bonus. Since the emancipation of women, the Western attitude in both sexes means partnerships or marriages where romantic love is the initial basis of the relationship. This changing importance of romantic love is highlighted in the currently successful musical *Fiddler on the Roof*, where Tevye, with five daughters to marry off, finds his girls want love matches only.

Within the context of our definitions of romantic love, we can see that the experiencing of this state of mind and body will not be so much a function of the age or sex of the individual as a function of the temperament and personality of the individual. For not everyone is capable of romantic love and, for that matter, not everyone wants it. For some people sexual relationship is a practical means of mutual outlet for either or both partners. For others, romantic love as we have defined it is only possible in extra-marital sexual relationships where the 'thrill of a first love' is renewed again and again in new partners or in the dangers and secrecy of adultery. Romantic love may also be experienced only in the youthful days, free from the responsibilities of parenthood, householding and the competitive existence of making a living that is self-sufficient.

For others, romantic love is more an aim than a realizable achievement. It is tied closely to the concept of an 'equal marriage', where the basic motto is 'we share everything'. Here the economic and social life are shared mutually so that argument about money and friends and leisure activities are rare, and points of disagreement on other matters are ironed out by reasonable discussion. Sexual intercourse is mutually satisfactory and sexual tension is equitably controlled. The thrill of a love affair is not allowed to disrupt the harmony of this 'ideal' marriage.

It would be unfair in this discussion if I did not declare my own attitude to romantic love, though I am not about to make any Frank Harris or Fanny Hill confessions on this account. Having experienced it, it would be wrong for me to deny that it can contribute to the individual appreciation of sexual experiences. However, I am also practical enough (the commonsense I mentioned in the introduction) to appreciate that sexual relationship based purely on romantic love is bound to fail. It will fail because the relationship is essentially one of ego satisfaction in an aura of unreality and not one of mutual inter-personal satisfaction in an atmosphere that is strictly terrestrial. It will fail all the more if it is the only basis on which a marriage is expected to be built.

While age as such does not determine the romantic content of marriage, it would be reasonable to assume that a couple who have been married and mating (or not married but mating) for many years are less likely to have 'romantic' sexuality. Familiarity with each other's physical attributes, repetition of techniques, distractions of family life like children and house problems and distractions of working life, for example, are unlikely to encourage or maintain the special dream of pleasure in which radiant imagination and empathy are closely intertwined. Whether the couple individually or together recognize the apathy of such a sexual relationship will depend to some extent on the momentum of their whole married (or mated) life. For many the inertia is so great that neither partner bothers to try and alter the setting or the technique. For some, they are roused from this inertia only by the spirit of romance in new or extra-marital contacts. For others either or both partners make renewed efforts to kindle the old flame in a change of technique and setting, which still fits in with their other activities of daily living. Such changes may well be more difficult to achieve in older people whose ageing has produced a conservative and narrowed outlook and a diminution in the general intensity of emotions.

There was a delightful television advertisement not so long ago that somehow parodied Charles Kingsley's famous saying that 'some say the age of chivalry is past and the spirit of romance is dead : never, so long as there is a wrong left unredressed on this earth'. In the advertisement a queen-like bride enters her new palace-like home in an aura of candle light and flowers. In a trice, however, she is sadly transformed into a Cinderella-like prisoner of greasy pots and pans piled high in the kitchen. How to release her so she can return to her queen-like state? Wash up, they tell us with their special brand of soap-filled steel wool and bring a shine of candle light back into the bride's life. I certainly do not recall Freud ever considering a soap-filled pad of steel wool as a romantic sex symbol. Yet the message of the soft sell is clear. Married life needs romance and woman needs her femininity.

Romantic love is reflected not only in the world of advertising but also in contemporary films, plays, books and pop songs. Marriage counsellors recognize their influence on the mating of couples who expect to 'fall in love'; they may do so, but then founder on the colder realities of living as two and not one. They admit the usefulness of romance in initial cohesion but encourage the cementing of the marriage framework with the more solid bonds of joint achievements and joint goals. As I have already indicated sexual activity can take place in an unromantic setting and without either of our definitions of romantic love, yet still relieve the sexual tensions of the partners. The romantic aura, when it is present, gives a nuance to the relationship whatever the age of the partners and however long that relationship has continued.

So we amend our fourth idea and acknowledge that 'romantic love occurs in the young and in the not-so-young'.

This brings us to our fifth link idea that one of the reasons for youth being a choice setting for sexual function is

the peak health of their sex (and other) organs. I said earlier that defining health is not easy, and for that matter,
defining peak health is even less easy. I once attended a
lecture by a distinguished professor of medicine entitled
'The Nature of Disease'. Many of us in the audience had
anticipated that this gifted doctor, famed for his diagnosis
and therapy of certain illnesses, would concentrate on his
'favourite illnesses'. We expected a long and high-powered
discussion on viruses and bacteria and on genetic theories
of susceptibility. Instead we were treated to a discourse in
semantics, an exercise in logic, and a somewhat philosophi-
cal conclusion that disease had best be viewed in the context
of the patient who was 'not at ease'. If I were to follow the
path of our professor of medicine, I might overcome the
difficulty of defining health by calling it 'being at ease', and
peak health 'being very much at ease'. Applied to physical
organs it sounds just a little odd, however, and we have to
fall back on the obvious definition of a healthy organ being
one that is doing its job regularly as required.

Thus we could describe the male and female sexual apparatus as being healthy if it can function regularly as
required. The idea of 'peak health' for an organ in terms of
its function is not quite physiological. Generally speaking
healthy body organs work at an optimum level though in
some cases – for example, kidneys and liver – there is a
reserve area 'in case of emergencies'. Such reserves would
only be mobilized if disease attacked the organs. We will
consider the male sexual organs later but at this juncture
we can acknowledge that healthy testicles and penis and an
intact healthy nerve-supply from brain to spinal cord to
the organs should permit erection and intercourse and emission if the sexual tension calls for that form of outlet. For
the female, a healthy vulva and vaginal canal with intact
healthy nerve-supply from brain to spinal cord to the canal
should permit intromission and relief of tension or full

orgasm if the sexual tension calls for that form of sexual outlet.

The general process of body ageing is a complex affair. It progresses at different rates for different individuals. It may be retarded by inherited factors, environment, nutrition and physical and mental activity. Alternatively it may be accelerated by the same factors of heredity and environment, by lack of suitable nutrition and by restriction of physical and mental activity. The advent of disease or illness in either sex, but particularly in the male, further accelerates ageing processes. In the case of the sexual organs the factors already mentioned still apply but there is added the effect of hormonal changes, particularly in the female sex. Sexual organ function is controlled not only by nerves from the brain and spinal cord but by chemical substances called hormones, secreted by the so-called ductless glands. As we shall again be considering later, in the female the levels of oestrogen hormone are particularly important in maintaining the health of the vulva and vagina and also the breasts. Oestrogen levels in any woman vary somewhat over the 'fertile period', that is from the first onset of the menstrual cycle to the menopause. After the menopause, there is generally a diminution in oestrogen levels but the level again varies from one woman to another. The ageing changes in the sex organs may consequently be little in one woman or marked in another. (The influence of psychological changes at the menopause may also be minor or major not adding, or adding, to mechanical difficulties of sexual function as the case may be.) These hormonal deficiency changes can be corrected by oestrogen medication, however, so that this kind of ageing is reversible.

In the male, the hormonal changes are much more gradual and failure of erection – the classical 'sign of ageing' – may be just as much the result of psychological problems as physical degeneration, even in the seventies. The effects

of (male) sex hormone (such as testosterone) are less pre-
dictable than in the female, however, once true ageing changes have occurred.

Our fifth link idea, then, has also to be amended. It might
now be phrased that 'sexual function at any age is feasible
if the sex organs are healthy, and there is no real peak
health that makes youth a more choice setting than later
years'. That sexual activity gives us our 'highest heights as
well as our deepest depths below' is true for youth as well
as for later life. Youth can never be a guarantee of a sexual
El Dorado.

Our discussions in the present and previous chapter have
shown us that the basis for sex being exclusively linked with
youth is none too solid. Yet the myth of minimal sex in
middle and later years is strong enough. Children of widowed or divorced 'older' parents sometimes look askance
when mum or dad takes up the social round again. They
often express surprise when mum or dad indicates an in-
tention to remarry, and eyebrows arch higher at the pros-
pect of the parent actually sleeping with the new partner.
Phrases like 'be your age, mum' are trotted out by the son
or daughter who cannot conceive how mum could love
anyone but their dad (the romantic notion again), and cannot accept the continuing sexual needs of older people. So
much for the progress of the younger generation in understanding the older generation!

The Right Diagnosis

Medical students learning to take a clinical history of a
patient are generally advised to give the patient 'the benefit
of the doubt'. In other words, in the first instance, if a
patient says he has a headache or backache, for example,
the medical student must accept this as being accurate and

truthful. In a sense, it is analogous to the training of shop assistants who are taught that the customer is always right. After he qualifies, the young doctor begins to learn how to judge the reliability of patients' statements about themselves and events in their lives. Both the family doctor and the hospital specialist develop their experience, so that they can determine if the symptoms are neurotic, or are hysterical, or are coloured by physical illness, or are inaccurate through fading memory or serious mental illness. If this is true for organic disturbance and mental problems, it is equally true for difficulties and disturbances in sexual life.

An understanding of the ideas already discussed and of several other factors can help the professional sex counsellor to assess the older client who seeks help. It also guides the physician whose help is sought for apparently non-sexual problems, if it seems appropriate. The right diagnosis may then be attempted and reached.

Two examples illustrate the point. A woman in her early forties was seen by her family doctor because she complained of headaches, dizziness, and loss of balance while up a ladder cleaning a window. The doctor examined her and found her blood pressure normal and nothing else physically amiss. He communicated his findings to the patient expecting her to be very grateful, but instead she burst into tears. With sympathetic questioning he elicited the true reason why the patient had come to see him. She was approaching the menopause, had never really enjoyed sexual relations with her husband, and had anticipated menopausal symptoms which she was using as an 'honourable' excuse to finish her sex life with her husband. A previously fit thirty-five-year-old labourer had an accident at a demolition site in which a metal bar struck his foot. He was wearing capped boots at the time so he had no actual fracture in the foot bones but much swelling and bruising. Not unreasonably he sought compensation and equally reason-

bly he was offered a small sum – apart from maintenance of wages – by the firm concerned. He saw his doctor and was referred to a specialist to whom he complained of headache, insomnia, aching in his whole leg and complete impotence with his attractive brunette wife. Further questioning elicited his feeling that the compensation being offered to him was insufficient considering the alleged effects on his health. With the patient's permission, his wife was interviewed. She confirmed that the accident had upset her husband a great deal but denied any failure in the sexual side of their marriage in the period after the accident.

In both these patients, accepting the symptoms and the story at face value would have prevented the doctors from moving towards the right diagnoses and giving the right advice and treatment. So also sex counsellors and those whose work involves them in solving sex problems need to learn how to elicit the essential factors in a client's or patient's sexual life. This applies equally to social workers and parents, to doctors and probation officers, to teachers and psychologists, for example, and is just as important when dealing with older people as when dealing with the young. In the case of older people, the tendency to view sexual matters in a resigned manner, with such phrases as 'at your age you cannot expect anything else', or, 'you must expect to lose your sexual feelings at the change of life', are consistent with the youth and sex, age and no sex, view we have previously discussed. They are unfortunate attitudes and may be unhelpful not only in being incorrect, but also in perpetuating the other faulty concept that old age is a disease.

The right diagnosis of sexual needs or problems in older people may be difficult to determine, not just because of natural embarrassment at discussing intimacies with 'strangers'. Older people may be afraid of seeming ridiculous or childishly immature or unwordly if they reveal their sexual interests, wants or dislikes. The real position may then never be revealed, or may be unintentionally brought to light by, for example, an extra-marital affair. Alternatively, the psycho-physical strains may be translated into physical complaints about organs remote from the sexual parts, as in our first example above.

Sexual customs in any given community are as varied as the faces of those who practise them. Many factors influence the form of sexual outlet for the single or married male or female. Both secular education and religious training can modify the physical forms of outlet and the associated emotional state. The example and influence of parents, of both the male and female partners, can limit or extend the expressions of their mutual sexual outlets. The social status of the partners, often tied up with their economic circumstances, can also affect the mode of sexual outlet. Basic personality traits such as being outgoing or introverted, also affect sexual outlet habits. The fact of being single or married, or widowed or divorced, must also bear weight on the psycho-physical expressions of sexual outlet. The possible permutations would require a computer to encompass all of them.

If an attempt were made to gauge, on top of the above information, what is normal for a given age and what is usual for a given state of health, sex counsellors could be in a better position to compare the general facts with the particular ones. The surveys of sexual practice made over the past four decades would then be of value not merely as of academic interest but in helping to make the right diagnosis. This right diagnosis would then be a preliminary to seeking a practical solution in a given case.

In order to reach the right diagnosis in older people, three other factors require consideration. Among such people discussion of sex has generally taken place in groups of women or of men but not in mixed company. This form of cultural taboo is now waning, especially in the younger generation. The attitudes among a group of men reflect the idea that older people are less active or inactive sexually, at least within the marriage setting. This is apparent from their after-dinner stories, dirty jokes and personal adventure tales, and in verbal attitudes to single and married women. It is familiar too from the general conversation of pubs and clubs. Especially among working-class groups the male partner is assumed to be dominant in the sex life of a couple.

The attitudes among groups of women likewise reflect the notion that sexuality is much diminished or absent in later years. The male partner may be assumed to be dominant in the sexual relationship or, with more emancipated women, an equally active partner in a relationship whose tempo and climatic rhythm she can influence not just in a passive way.

Then there is the question of the physical health of either sexual partner. A number of illnesses appear in middle age which can affect the individual for long or short periods. Diseases such as bronchitis, heart complaints, and arthritis may produce a variety of physical changes with minor or major disabilities. With any illness there is an emotional aspect and this too varies from minor emotional upsets to major mental distress on a wide scale. Both physical and mental upsets can influence the sexual function of either or both partners. Sexual outlet may be voluntarily limited by a lowered sexual tension or by worry that sexual activity may worsen the physical illness. Caution in sexual activity may be recommended, by the doctor for the same reason.

In men there lingers an old superstition, moreover, that too frequent sexual outlet permanently weakens the human body. There is no scientific basis at all for this idea. It seems to have arisen from the notion that the semen emitted at ejaculation has an intrinsic life-sustaining quality, something like blood as it were, only 'stronger' because it contains the life force of unborn children in the sperm. The loss of such vital material would then weaken the body of the male losing it.

In fact the only real effect of having frequent sexual intercourse over, say, a forty-eight hour period, is a diminishing sperm count in the seminal fluid. This is not surprising when it is realized that the body manufactures two hundred million to six hundred million sperms for every two to four millilitres of ejaculated fluid. Fortunately, the physiological manufacturing process, given twenty-four hours rest, quickly gears up again to return the sperm count to normal levels again for the next supply of ejaculate.

The social position of the older single man or woman, whether unmarried, widowed or divorced, is more sensitive in terms of sexual outlet than his or her married contemporaries. If the group attitude towards the older single person denies such a person the 'right' to continued sexual outlet, and assumes such a person has no sexual needs, this may encourage guilt feelings in single older people when they do have sexual tension and relieve it by some form of sexual activity. The feeling of guilt may be greater if the outlet is masturbatory (a form of outlet formerly regarded as 'sinful') rather than in erotic wet dreams (which are somehow beyond voluntary 'control').

Redressing the Balance

In this book so far we have indicated that there is a faulty understanding of sexual tension and of the need for sexual outlet in the middle and later years of what we have called 'the longer life'. Associated with this imperfect knowledge are mistaken attitudes towards sex in later life – attitudes which can be distressing to those who wish to enjoy or might otherwise enjoy the expressions of sexuality in their single or married life. The improvement of our understanding about sex in later years, and a corresponding enlightenment of attitudes, is not a simple matter of providing the right information and leaving the person who has been so informed to draw his or her own conclusions. The behaviour of individuals and groups in a given social environment, as revealed in a sociological survey, may prove to be unacceptable to other individuals or groups of a different cultural and ethnic background or of a different age setting or of a different social class. Similarly the forms of sexual outlet and the pattern of sexual behaviour revealed in a sexological survey in, say, the Polynesian Islands, may be of academic or erotic interest to the young marrieds at a suburban night school sociology course. The adoption of these forms of outlet and behaviour in their own sex lives, however, is unlikely, because of their differing patterns of education, upbringing, social role, moral law and urban environment.

Nevertheless, awareness of other practices in sexual outlet and other attitudes towards sexual tension can influence the informed group in the long run. Such influence may be felt sooner in a society like our own Western civilization, where the social order is changing and where there is a parallel break-up in family and ethnic traditions. For in such a state of flux, both individuals and groups are willing to experiment with various patterns of conduct in order to try to find a widely acceptable way of life that will again produce stability and emotional wellbeing. Such experimentation may be a haphazard taking up and setting down of ideas and practices, or a more rational sorting out of those practices and ideas which have undesirable consequences for the individual or group, from those which will be of benefit in both the short and the long term. For example, if it is clear that promiscuous sexual intercourse raises the venereal disease rate in the community, there is a good argument for discouraging such promiscuity even if the sexual behaviour itself promotes emotional wellbeing. If, on the other hand, for example, the venereal disease rate is actually low and is readily controlled by antibiotic drugs, there is no real argument against promiscuous sexual intercourse if it promotes emotional wellbeing. If yet again it is shown that promiscuous sexual intercourse undermines group social stability although promoting emotional wellbeing for some individuals, this would be a long-term reason for opposing it.

In view of the complex factors which affect sexual development in any individual and determine both the levels of sexual tension and the forms of sexual outlet, it is important to recognize in any individual what sexual patterns represent deviations within the wide range of normal, and what represents the product of a psychotically disturbed or psychopathic personality. Thus, for example, a couple which indulges in spanking of one or other partner as a preliminary means of arousal prior to sexual intercourse can be considered within the normal deviations, whereas a partner who achieves sexual outlet merely in the spanking itself, without requiring sexual intercourse, can be regarded as an abnormal deviant.

Thus, to begin redressing the balance of sexuality in older people, we must be aware of the levels of sexual tension and of the forms of outlet in individuals and groups. We must try to sort out the consequences of such behaviour in terms of stabilizing the sexual function and emotional wellbeing of the older age groups. Moreover, we must be on guard against deviations of sexual behaviour which are the product of mental illness or mental instability. Further, as we have seen in the last chapter, we should attempt to reach the right diagnosis when sexual problems arise in older people and this requires both the broader knowledge of sexual behaviour and a fuller interest in the physiological and pathological changes of the older mind and body.

The following story illustrates these points. A district nurse, leaving the house of a patient, was stopped by a somewhat agitated middle-aged lady whom she did not know but who asked her if she could speak on a personal matter. She followed the lady into her home and no sooner had she closed the door than the lady anxiously inquired how she could tell if her sixty-two year old husband was being unfaithful? The lady showed the nurse a pair of the husband's underpants and pointed to some obvious seminal stains as presumptive evidence of his infidelity. This was underlined by an explanation that her husband had lost interest in loveplay and sexual intercourse with her over the previous three months, and this despite such efforts to arouse him as the recent purchase of a transparent négligée. The physical health of husband and wife was sound and he was active at work and in his social life. She had experienced the menopause ten years before this with little physical or emotional upset.

The district nurse, herself a married woman in her forties, was used to requests for advice of a non-nursing nature in the course of her duties. The plea for help in this sexual problem was somewhat disconcerting, however, for she was surprised that this older couple had actually been enjoying sexual relations in their sixth decade. Even more surprising to her was the wife's anxiety to continue these sexual relations, expressed in the suspicion that her husband was taking his favours elsewhere, and in her efforts to stimulate his desire. What the district nurse did not consider was the fact that this fifty-eight year old wife saw her as an authority figure upon whom she could call for advice. Further, she would take the nurse's advice as correct simply because it came from a figure of authority in her community.

Sex and the Longer Life

While it is relatively easy to advance the sexual education of a professional group like district nurses or doctors, by introducing lectures, discussions and data in film or book form to their educational syllabus, it is very much harder to disseminate the facts and ideas on sex in older people to a non-captive audience. Books such as this one, magazines and newspapers that publish in depth, television and films in the documentary or didactic vein, can all be used. From the point of view of older people, the spread of facts and advice on sex in later life can be incorporated in preventive health projects. These latter may be undertaken by private specialist bodies, such as the Institute of Directors preventive health centres, or the project begun by Rutherglen local authority in the early 1950s that has been taken up by other local authorities, in the form of preventive health clinics for the over-fifty-fives. At these preventive clinics, executives and other working individuals (housewives included) are referred for medical check-ups and appropriate X-rays or blood tests. The doctors at these clinics can then offer advice on diet, exercise, working conditions, medical therapy and other measures to maintain or improve fitness at middle and later ages. To these could be added advice on sexual needs and problems where required or when requested. This assumes that doctors running these clinics will themselves have the knowledge and training in sexual matters that would be required.

Another educative outlet for the spread of information on sex in older people could be the pre-retirement courses of local authorities or individual employing groups. With the advent of the longer life (both longer working life and longer retired life), much interest has been generated in preparing people of all social groups and classes of employment for the period running up to and after retirement. The effects of retirement in the male, on his community and domestic status, on his income, on his social life, on his personality and outlook, have been studied, and suitable approaches to the practical considerations of retirement and leisure have been worked out. This applies, if less dramatically, to the female. Generally speaking, however, attendance at the talks and films in the pre-retirement courses, and consideration of the books published on retirement problems of men and women, give virtually no hint that sexual tension and sexual outlet might be worthy of attention. Philosophy, often sugary, sometimes cynical, is for the ageing, but certainly not carnality.

Since professional counsellors such as psychiatrists, medical social workers and geriatricians, for example, are available if not actually lecturing in these courses, it would help to redress the balance if formal lectures and informal discussions on sex in later life could be included in the syllabus. The 'mixed groups' taboo need not be a problem at discussion time as separate courses are held for men and for women, as a rule.

The special role of the marriage guidance counsellor will be discussed later. In fact, any member of the groups of professional social workers, such as health visitors, social welfare workers, probation officers, can be educated in the facts of sex in older people to the further benefit of those whose problems they come into contact with, and those to whom they give help on a professional or voluntary basis.

As a distinguished health visitor emphasized at a national conference on preventive health education, those whose work involves them in any form of health education must learn to 'un-teach' ideas that are based on illogicalities and wrong assumptions. This is an essential preliminary to any individual or group programme designed to impart clearer appreciation and encourage better methods of maintaining and improving health. This idea of 'un-teaching' applies equally in the area of sex education for those who have the benefit of a longer life.

c

2 | The Changing Body

Defining the Phase of Life

The reader will have noted from the chapter headings in this book that, in undertaking to discuss the changes in later life which are especially relevant to sexual function, the third and fourth chapters appear to separate changes in the body from changes in the mind. Such a firm separation of mind and body is not in keeping with our current understanding of human make-up. The study of psychosomatic medical complaints, such as peptic ulcer for example, vividly illustrates the constant interaction of mind upon body activities and of body on mental activities. Therefore any firm separation of mind and body changes in middle and old age is an artificial one, used only where it seems appropriate to clarify a particular problem or situation. In fact, throughout the present and subsequent chapters, the mutual influence of psyche and soma will be considered under either heading.

In discussing the physical and mental changes in sexual function in that part of the longer life known as middle age and old age, it should be helpful to define just what we mean by middle age and old age. It is interesting that although we use these terms for stages in our life cycle so readily in our daily conversation, their definition in strict scientific criteria is not easy. There are several lines along which a definition might run. These include the actual number of years a given individual has lived, and the physical appearance of that individual. They also include an assessment of the physical strength and of the mental wellbeing, and of the effects of disease in that individual. Further, a definition may involve the attitude of the social or ethnic group to which the individual belongs, as well as the personal attitude of the individual towards himself, his surroundings and his contemporaries.

Taking the actual number of years lived, as a reference point for middle age and old age, an arbitrary range might be forty-five to sixty-five for middle age and sixty-five onwards for old age. This assumes a longer life span than the statistical life expectation at birth of seventy-two years.

Using chronological age as a marker also ignores the variation in rate of physical and psychological change in the individual, which may be faster or slower than his or her contemporaries. Further, it discounts the wide variations in the social role and career level of individuals enjoying similar social roles and pursuing similar careers. For one may be, for example, a grandmother at thirty-five, forty-five, or fifty-five, or a director joining the board at thirty, forty, or fifty.

Again, if we take the physical appearance of the individual as a marker for the middle age and old age phases, we find that thinning and greying of the hair allegedly indicate middle age and baldness old age, or that facial wrinkling and 'double' chins indicate middle age, and neck wrinkling and loss of skin sheen old age. Once again, however, a number of factors create wide variations in the outward appearance and physical state of individuals at given chronological age. Ill health for example can affect the physical appearance adversely. The common anaemia of women due to iron deficiency causes skin pallor, lethargic attitude, and a drawn expression, while thyroid gland deficiency produces dry skin, scalp hair loss, and a puffy expression. The former illness may 'age' a woman's external appearance by five to ten years while the latter can make a thirty-year-old look like a woman in her sixties. Exercise, or lack of it, similarly affects the physique. The desk-bound clerk, whose evening entertainment is television and whose weekend relaxation is a drive in the car, may lose the tone of his abdominal muscles, producing a middle-age spread while he is well under forty. The executive who keeps fit in the gymnasium and on the golf course can walk and sit erectly and move with firm strides, belying an age in the middle sixties. Inherited factors can also play a part. Not only may longevity be passed on – the grandparents who survive to their eighties genetically encourage the grandchildren to survive similarly into their eighties – but youthful appearance in later life may also be passed on through the generations. At the other extreme, the rare condition of accelerated abnormal ageing in a child, called progeria, may also be the result of genetic disturbance. Climate, too, can affect the external physical appearance although the relationship is not always clear. Persistent exposure to the drying and weathering effects of sun and wind may alter the facial appearance and the appearance of other skin areas exposed, sometimes producing a premature ageing effect. Certain climatic areas – usually remote from civilization – such as Georgia on the Russo-Turkish border, are claimed as encouraging longevity and youthful physical appearance. This is based on the apparently high number of active centenarians in such regions. Closer examination may reveal defective evidence in terms of vital statistics, overlaid with the subconscious desire to discover a shangri-la on our planet. Similarly, the physical strength at any age will be affected by occupation, natural endowment, frequency of exercise, ill health and climatic conditions, for example.

The mental wellbeing of the individual can provide an important clue to middle age and old age. If we exclude actual disease of the brain from organic illness, or the severe mental illnesses such as schizophrenia and depressive psychosis, the mental outlook and the mental performance of the individual can be helpful in plotting the phase he or she belongs to. Thus the middle-aged individual sees himself or herself as still in the mainstream of daily life, as having achieved some ambitions but still having more to aim for, as no longer being radical merely for the sake of being rebellious, as no longer being interested exclusively in the current activities of 'young people', and as being able to make a retrospective self-assessment as well as a prospective one. The individual in old age sees himself or herself moving slowly onwards from the previous mental outlook to a partial disengagement from mainstream activities, to a transfer of goals from ambition to personal satisfaction and comfort, to a readjustment to the social and economic conditions of retirement.

As I have said, not only mental outlook but mental performance gives some guide to the life cycle stage. Thus middle age finds the individual quite capable of coping with routine procedures, simple or complex, and yet able to tackle new situations and new problems on the basis of past experience and intelligent adjustment. The potential level of performance, however, may be less than when he or she was younger and capable of faster organization of his or her mental processes. While old age may or may not find the individual quite capable of coping with routine procedures, simple or complex, the ability to tackle new situations and new problems has diminished and there is a decline in operative flexibility, confidence and efficiency in these new situations. Again, other factors such as intelligence quotient, occupational skill, illness and inherent creativity will modify the generalized picture of mental performance that I have outlined.

Two physical changes which are sometimes used as markers for middle age and old age respectively are presbyopia and shuffling gait. Presbyopia is a defect in vision which commonly appears in the forties and results in the need to wear spectacles for reading small print. Shuffling or slow measured gait refers to the method of walking in many older people. It is by no means universal but does contrast with the brisker walking pace of young people, and is a reflection of some loss of confidence in independent loco-motion.

Another physical marker, in the female human being, which is often taken as the starting point of middle age is the menopause. This is a satisfactory pointer in chrono-logical terms, provided the menopause is a 'natural' one and not induced by illness or gynaecological operation in the thirties, for example. Even then, 'natural' menopause does occur in some young women who are clearly not middle-aged. Nevertheless, as we shall discuss shortly in this chapter, the menopause in women does have a distinct physical and psychological bearing on sex function in middle age, as well as on general health, personality and outlook.

The state provides a fiscal marker to retirement, if not officially to old age, by awarding the retirement pension to women at sixty and men at sixty-five. But not many house-wives retire at sixty, and not every worker begins his or her retirement at sixty-five or sixty respectively. So its useful-ness as an old age marker is only relative to the need for a welfare state to choose a demarcation line for its support of older people.

From what we have said, it emerges that there is no easy all-embracing definition of middle age and of old age. In a given individual or in a given group of persons, however, there are a number of objective clues and subjective point-ers which help us to establish the individual or group in the middle-age or old-age phase of the life cycle.

The Female Menopause

It is an interesting fact that women, describing the functions or illnesses of the female body to other women or in 'mixed' company, very often employ euphemisms. For example, painful menstruation is being 'unwell', operation for removal of the womb is 'operation for a woman's complaint', and even being pregnant is to be 'expecting'. Presumably this verbal delicacy of expression dates back to unemancipated womanhood and the days of 'feminine mystery', those former times, for example, when the family doctor delivered the baby under the modest cover of bedclothes or, even worse, was allowed to attend the delivery only after the baby was born.

While euphemisms in medicine play a useful role in allaying fears and anxiety – the malignant tumour sounds less formidable as a 'lump' or a 'growth' – the use of euphemisms in normal healthy human functions may encourage the opposite effect. If being 'unwell' paraphrases menstruation, the woman who is menstruating is encouraged to feel literally unwell. The female menopause is popularly called the 'change of life'. This phrase could be argued as fair and truthful and not particularly euphemistic, for the complete cessation of monthly menstruation is certainly a change in the previous way of life. But if you consider the menopause from the physiological aspect, that is, the end of fertility and capacity for reproduction in the woman at her menopause, then 'change of life' is one of those undesirable euphemisms which invite anxiety and misunderstanding.

Climacteric is an alternative word for menopause, implying a critical moment in the female life as if the balance of mind and body is hovering at the brink. While this is a dramatic expression of the physical and psychological changes which do or may occur, I prefer the term menopause as being realistic without being sinister.

A medical teacher of my student days used to talk about menstruation as the 'weeping of a disappointed womb' for, as a physiologist, he regarded pregnancy as the 'natural' state of fertile womanhood. The monthly bleeding, in which the womb discards the nourishing lining prepared for a fertilized ovum, has its onset or menarche in girls from about thirteen onwards. The menopause marks the final point in the recurring monthly cycle of womb preparation and discarding. It may be a sudden or gradual cessation of menstruation at any time from the start of the forties to the beginning of the fifties. Generally speaking, the younger a woman starts menstruating, the older she is when she finishes – and not, as might have been expected, the sooner she finishes. In a few women, a natural menopause occurs earlier, in the thirties. Certain illnesses, for example disease of the pituitary gland, and certain medical treatments, for example surgical removal of the ovaries and radiotherapy of the ovaries, can produce an 'artificial' menopause at any age in the fertile years.

The basic cause of the natural menopause is a decline in the function of the ovaries, which stop producing ova for fertilization and which stop producing the oestrogen hormone. If no ova are produced, fertility is absent as no embryo can be created by fertilization. This loss of fertility occurs at an age – middle age – when, as we have noted, a good deal of introspection and self-assessment is going on. The reaction to the fact that she can no longer produce children varies from one woman to the next. For example, if the middle-aged woman in marriage is already perturbed by the loss of her motherly role with her children gone from the fold, the menopausal loss of fertility may accentuate her feeling of being 'useless' to the family. If the middle-aged woman who is single but always felt she might one day marry and have a family is already feeling the demarcation from youth and its higher potential for marriage, the menopausal loss of fertility may underline her position in an uncomfortable way. If the middle-aged married woman has been the mother of a large family but has been looking forward to more social freedom, the fertility loss is viewed with equanimity and a start may be made for directing her time and energy in new directions.

To these reactions are added the effects of a drop in oestrogen hormone production, and these effects can be both physical and psychological. Oestrogen does influence mental outlook and the physical wellbeing of all women. The extent to which deprivation of this hormone affects mind and body varies considerably from one woman to another. This is true both for the variations within the menstrual cycle of each woman in her fruitful years, and the actual fall in hormonal level which occurs at the menopause. The variation in the actual fall in hormone levels from one menopausal woman to another helps to determine why one woman sails through the menopause with minimal physical or mental upset, another has considerable mind and body upset, and a third has only moderate mental or physical symptoms and signs. This means that 'the menopause' is as individual as the woman in whom it occurs and there is no fixed or 'normal' pattern which can be expected.

Oestrogen hormone influences the development and changes in the breasts and in the vagina and womb. The hormone also influences the nourishment of the skin and smooth muscle and appears to have a 'protective' influence against circulatory diseases up to middle age. Thus a sharp fall in oestrogen hormone levels or a drop in already low levels of oestrogen can interfere with the nourishment of the body parts already mentioned. The hormone also influences mental outlook so that a fall in oestrogen levels can produce either 'new' mental symptoms, such as headache or irritability or sleeplessness, or even depression, or exaggerate 'old' mental instabilities such as nervousness and anxiety. By new and old, I mean new to the individual's mental state and personality, and old if there have always been mental problems. These, then, are the physical and mental changes with which the middle-aged woman, already reconsidering her role as mother, wife, sexual partner, career woman and citizen, has to contend.

The medical attitude to the menopause was firstly a conservative one, in which the menopause was seen as a natural law of womanhood that should not be disturbed. Later, it was considered reasonable therapy to treat the physical and mental symptoms which did occur with small doses of synthetic oestrogens for limited periods of time. Sedatives were also given for the mental symptoms, and full psychiatric treatment in menopausal depression.

We have already looked at the many factors which influence sexual tension and modify sexual needs and outlet in any one individual. If middle age is a time for looking back and looking forward in self-appraisal, the sexual 'state' of the woman may also be included in her personal reflections. In the case of the married woman, if the marriage is stabilized and sexual outlets are within the marriage, sexual tension is fairly fixed in its level. These levels may be lesser or greater than in younger years according to how much sexual enjoyment and satisfaction, personal and mutual, has altered with the years. In the case of the single woman, either unmarried or separated, divorced or widowed, here too the level of sexual tension is fairly stable (provided enough time has elapsed from the loss of the 'fixed' partner) and the mode of outlet is reasonably fixed in its pattern.

The arrival of the menopause with its small or large degree of physical and psychological changes is very likely to affect sexual tension and, to a lesser extent, the sexual outlet. There may be a minor or major fall in sexual tension with corresponding loss of interest in sexual outlet. In some women, there is contrastingly a rise in sexual tension, which is variously explained as being due to 'not having to worry about pregnancies' or being due to 'fear of the husband looking elsewhere because of loss of his wife's youthful charms' or because of the 'need to resume a more wifely role now that motherhood is clearly over'.

For the male partner, too, middle age is a time of re-assessment and reflection. Whether single or married, he may experience an upsurge in sexual tension as he compares himself with younger men and feels the former urge to compete for the sexual outlet of (often younger) other women. Alternatively, as we shall discuss in a moment, he too may experience menopausal symptoms in late middle age, although these are far from the clear-cut female changes, and his sexual tensions and outlet may be diminished. In either case, the clash with the problems of his female partner can rock the most stable of relationships and splinter those which are already shaky. It requires time, advice, support and therapy to ride out the difficulties and re-establish relationships where possible. The point that must be stressed in terms of sex in the longer life is this: the female menopause, with its cessation of menstruation and involution in the function of the ovaries, need not and does not also imply the cessation of sexual tension and the regression of sexual outlet in middle-aged women.

The Male Menopause

There is an interesting phenomenon known as couvade, in which the husband of a pregnant woman apparently experiences some of her 'discomforts'. He may complain, for example, of heartburn or backache or fancies for certain foods. These complaints are resolved when his wife has been delivered of the baby. They are an example of psycho-physical sympathy in an intense interpersonal relationship of man and wife. It is my own theory that the features of the male menopause which resemble those of the female menopause do so because of an analogous, but not identical, sympathetic interpersonal bond. Of course, men neither menstruate nor ovulate, so that loss of fertility and lack of oestrogen hormone cannot play any part in a male menopause. Some doctors in fact deny that there is any comparable phase in men like the female menopause. They say truthfully that middle age in men is just as much a time for self-appraisal in prospective and retrospective terms, so that anxiety, headache and irritability are the result of looking back at lost causes and opportunities and looking forward to further problems, occupational, domestic and health.

In the middle-aged man, changes in sexual tension with a reduction in sexual interest and outlet may occur. Alternatively, there may be an upsurge in sexual interest. In married men this is often directed towards extra-marital outlets, and in both single and married men directed towards younger women. These alterations in sexual levels may be part of the steadily declining sexual tension and outlet in an individual male, seen from the historical view of his life. They are not related to changes in sex gland or male hormone function as these normally continue into the seventh or even eighth decade. Both a decline and an upsurge may be the result of the problems of middle age, in terms of social and marital status, self-reflection on physical state and the relations with the usual sex partner. Thus one man may feel bored or frustrated with his job, upset at the state of his marriage, troubled by some real or problematical illness and bothered that he is no longer attractive to other women.

Another man may feel secure and happy in his job, stable

in his state of marriage, not especially bothered by health worries, but no longer excited or stimulated in the familiarity of his sexual outlet with his wife. A third man, reasonably safe and moderately interested in his job, single by non-marriage or separation or widowerhood, probably somewhat introspective towards his health, may continue with his own mode of sexual outlet but notices he is less interested or less easily aroused. Such a cross-section of 'case histories' allows us to anticipate differing attitudes and responses in the sexual part of this middle-age phase. For example, the first man might separate from or divorce his wife and take up a new partner. The second man might seek extra-marital 'stimulation' or continue as before. The third man may answer an advertisement in a magazine offering improvement in sexual arousal by drugs or appliances, or turn to a new partner. Both the life patterns and the sexual adjustments are, of course, infinitely more variable than the three examples I have given.

As with the female menopause, the alteration in sexual tension must not be taken as necessarily permanent and implying an early cessation in sexual tension and outlet.

The Medical Flaws

One of the perennial arguments against medical therapy in connexion with the human body is the suggestion that it 'interferes with nature'. Closer examination of the circumstances in which this argument is used often reveals a personal interest in maintaining the *status quo* for social, emotional or financial reasons. Even if it is proposed on religious grounds in a sincere setting, the idea of not interfering with physical and mental changes in the human body is still more likely to be based on an irrational or superstitious fear of the consequences than on a logically

conceived, scientifically assessed estimate of the likely out-
come. The history of smallpox vaccination, using Jenner's
cowpox vaccine, is a good example. Smallpox as a plague
ravaged these islands until voluntary vaccination with cowpox was introduced. As people argued that vaccination
interfered with nature and areas remained unimmunized
because of defaulters, government legislation made vaccination and quarantine compulsory. This public health measure
ended the terror of massive smallpox outbreaks and 'nature'
was successfully reversed. Later, in the calm of a smallpox-
free population, Parliament became concerned with the freedom of the individual (to choose medical care) and the Act
of compulsory vaccination was rescinded. Today we have an
uneasy compromise between an under-vaccinated population and occasional outbreaks of smallpox.

At least with infectious diseases, however, we can always
argue that the organisms invading the body are unnatural
and should therefore be resisted by medical therapy. In the
case of physiological changes, such as pregnancy or the
menopause, the great 'nature' cry is re-invoked.

While some lay people and some doctors in the earlier
part of this century feared that effective birth control by
male rubber condom or female rubber cap would encourage wild promiscuity and widespread venereal disease – at
least so they expressed themselves in print – other doctors
and lay people welcomed this effort at population control
on a national and on a personal level. The coming of the
female birth-control pill has again roused the 'interfering
with nature' cry and, with it, the usual warnings of the dire
consequences to posterity as well as to the taker of the
pills. At least in the case of the condom, the anti-pill bri-
gade may say, it was an external block on natural conception and (presumably more important) it allowed the male
partner to take the decision of control or conception. Now
the women, via their doctors, are interfering with the regular

biological functions and hormonal control of their ovaries and, by themselves, can determine conception or control. Further, in the hands of the unmarried girl or woman, the pill is an effective aid to promiscuous enjoyment of sexual intercourse. In short, the family in society is in serious danger, both now and in coming generations, if the 'leave nature alone' group are to be believed. On balance, however, assuming the parallel with previous methods of birth control, women are likely to use the pill on an ever increasing scale and to fit its use, both inside and outside marriage, into their reassessed social status and social needs. The pill has certain unwanted side-effects such as nausea or fluid retention or – possibly – increased clotting tendency. These are likely to be eliminated as drug research and development improve the oestrogen-progestogen drugs in the pill. Some doctors still have nagging doubts that giving these hormones over many years might affect other hormone glands – pituitary and adrenal cortex, for example – but at the time of writing there is no conclusive evidence of any persistent detrimental effects.

Women taking oestrogenic birth-control pills who continue doing so into the late forties and early fifties have been found to suffer fewer or even no symptoms and physical changes of the menopause. This does not mean that the woman remains fertile and capable of conception – the ovaries regress and stop producing ova between forty-five and fifty whatever hormones she is having. The point is that the anxiety, irritableness, headache, skin changes, breast and vaginal changes do not occur. The psychophysical changes of this kind are avoided partly or completely. At the present time, however, doctors in this country recommend that from the age of forty-two onwards women who are taking birth-control pills should stop them for a few months at a time and use mechanical and/or chemical contraception. There are several reasons for this. In the first place, the doctor may be unable to assess whether the woman is having her menopause as she will continue menstruating as long as she is on the birth pill. Taking her off the pill will show if the periods are absent or diminishing. In the second place, there is the problem of diagnosis in the unsuspected cancer of the neck of the womb which sometimes arises at this age. This usually reveals itself by irregular bleeding but such evidence is suppressed by the 'regularizing' birth-control pill. Cancer of the neck of the womb has its highest incidence in married women before the menopause. It is suggested that the oestrogenic hormone may be either a predisposing or a stimulating factor in such cancerous growths. Many gynaecologists deny, however, that there is any real evidence in human females that oestrogens provoke or prosper malignancy in the womb. They suggest that menstruation is a protective factor in clearing potentially alterable tissue from the womb. They argue that in the healthy woman whose periods were regular on the pill there is less likelihood of womb cancer than in the general female population not on the pill.

At this juncture it is worth remembering that oestrogens are produced not only by the ovaries but also by the adrenal cortex. The latter does not cease functioning until death and is not affected by the menopause. Some women can therefore compensate their ovarian oestrogen loss at the menopause from the adrenal source. Such women maintain a more youthful appearance of skin and breasts and somewhat healthier genital tracts than their oestrogen-deficient counterparts. This higher oestrogen level means a low level of menopausal symptoms and much less likelihood of disturbed or difficult sexual relations. Progestogens are produced by the adrenal cortex as well as by the ovary. The need for extra progestogen therapy also varies according to how well the adrenal output compensates for the ovarian loss.

The gynaecologists who deny cancer-provoking properties of oestrogen are prepared to encourage its use. Either
as an oestrogen-progestogen single pill or as separate
oestrogen and progestogen therapy given in a 'natural' se-
quence, they advise commencing it well before the menopause and carrying it on through the expected menopausal
phase. The symptoms and physical changes, as I have noted
earlier, will be absent or reduced in the menopausal phase.
Further, enthusiasts for this therapy have noted that if this
oestrogen and progestogen treatment is continued on into the
sixties – with artificial menstruation as the sign that it is
hormonally effective – the woman maintains the physical
and emotional bloom of younger menstruating fertile women, yet does not have to worry about pregnancy.

Screening clinics run by the Public Health departments
of many towns are designed to detect disease in men and
women at the earliest, most treatable, stage. Thus such illnesses as tuberculosis (mass X-ray campaign) and sugar
diabetes have been discovered in screened groups. The examination of a cervical smear taken from the womb to
screen the cells for possible early malignant change, has
gained popularity among doctors and gynaecologists interested in cancer detection. The number of such screening
tests at special clinics has steadily increased. The same
technique – quick and painless for the woman, accurate for
the doctor – can be used to assess the level of oestrogen
activity on the female genital tract before, during and after
the menopause. Examination of womb cells under the mic-
roscope can confirm the external changes of oestrogen deficiency in the 'normal' women. This sort of assessment – of
the need for menopausal or post-menopausal oestrogen
hormones to improve and prolong feminine vigour and
sparkle – could be done at the Family Planning Clinic or
by the family doctor if the need for this was generally accepted.

Sex and the Longer Life

At a well-known geriatric preventive and screening clinic in the south of England, oestrogen therapy for older women has been provided by the medical director, and he reports clinical and photographic evidence of improvement in physical tone, health and appearance in the women attending the clinic. Sex function was also improved as the woman's physical and emotional state changed for the better.

While the conservative medical attitude remains one of 'leave the menopause alone', those gynaecologists on both sides of the Atlantic who advocate indefinite hormonal therapy into old age are steadily increasing. At a recent gynaecology symposium in a famous school of medicine, this form of replacement therapy was put forward strongly by one of the main speakers.

Another point is worth mentioning. The absence of a womb has no bearing on the hormone question although it can influence sexuality and sex function. The ultimate proof of this lies in those congenitally unfortunate girls who are born without a vagina (and without a womb). If they wish to have sexual intercourse, modern plastic surgery can provide a satisfactory artificial 'new' vagina, and the records show that subsequent sexual intercourse can be satisfactory for the girl and her male partner. The presence of ovaries or of adequate oestrogen hormone ensures the other aspects of femininity and, if she is married, adoption of children can complete her fulfilment.

Before leaving the question of the birth-control pill, the menopause and middle-age factors, it has been noted recently by some workers in the contraceptive research field that the pill itself can produce headache, irritability, restlessness and a decrease in sexual tension and desire for outlet. These are the very symptoms of the menopause itself although they are occurring in any age group of the females taking the pill. This is evidence which could dissuade doctors who are otherwise impressed by the helpful effect of oestrogens over the menopausal phase from continuing the pill into the fifties and sixties. Other medical reports in the official journals, however, have noticed a contrasting increase in sexual desire in some women. This conflict or apparent conflict of results shows once again that, at least in terms of sexual tension, the influence of psychological factors is very strong indeed whatever the drug therapy used.

The Masculine Cause

The point springs to mind that if modern hormone therapy and modern sex counselling assume female sexuality and sex function being carried on well into the post-menopausal years, then the masculine 'cause' must also be supported. I have considered the male menopause and indicated that sexual tensions and sexual outlet may or do persist into the seventies and even eighties in the male. In medical practice, the oldest cohabiting couple of whom I had personal knowledge were a man of ninety and his eighty-three-year-old wife. Attending for medical reasons, the wife confided that she thought it was 'really time they gave this up' but admitted that it was not difficult and it kept her husband happy. I sensed that, as they lived in an old people's bungalow, she was perturbed lest her neighbours knew they were still 'happily married'.

If that is thought of as an extreme example, the fact that men are capable of siring their own children while in their late seventies or even eighties is well authenticated and generally accepted. Examination of semen in such elderly men may show thinning of the ejaculate, which is due to reduction in the contributory fluids from the prostate gland and the seminal vesicles – parts that tend to thicken and scar with ageing. The total content of the ejaculate, which may be four millilitres in the younger male, may be reduced to one or two millilitres in the older man. Examination of the sperms shows reduction in numbers but many are still motile and viable and potentially capable of fertilization in the 'right environment'. In terms of sperm production, then, males may be potent until the eighth decade.

The testicles of the male produce the male hormone, testosterone. This male sex hormone promotes the pubertal growth and maintains the function (and size) of the fluid-producing seminal vesicles and prostate and the functional organ, the penis. Testosterone is, moreover, chemically concerned in erection of the penis and in determining ejaculation of the erect organ. This hormone is also responsible for the voice change at adolescence from enlargement of the larynx ('Adam's apple'). Proof of the effects of testicular hormone has been shown both in animal experiments and in the treatment with testosterone of under-developed boys with defective testicles. Not only do the latter's sex organs enlarge and become functional, but general muscular strength and sexual tensions and needs increase considerably. The lethargy and apathetic personality of the under-developed boy improves in an all-round sense. This infers that the emotional make-up and temperament of the male is dependent largely on testosterone.

If the testicles regress, thicken and diminish in function gradually over many years then the reduced level of testosterone results in general weakness and apathy. There is loss of sexual desire and sexual tensions, difficulties in erection and ejaculation, and nervous manifestations such as anxiety and irritability and even depression. Several workers have described this as the male climacteric (male menopause) and, drawing a parallel with the female run-down of hormones at the female menopause, suggested that the giving of testosterone should reduce the symptoms and improve well-being. This testicular regression is described as occurring in the late sixties and early seventies, that is ten to fifteen years after the average female menopause. This would suggest that the female biological clock is set to run down more quickly than the male clock – a fact which is not borne out by the statistical evidence of the much longer female life. Other workers have suggested that this testicular run-down is due to diminished blood-flow in the testicular arteries. The arteries, branches of the great aorta blood vessel, are affected by hardening and narrowing (arteriosclerosis) just like the rest of the body arteries. The testicles poorly supplied with blood cannot produce the previous levels of testosterone. This is quite a different process from the ovarian shut-down at the menopause. Moreover, the brain, heart and muscles are affected by the arteriosclerosis, and thus loss of potency, sexual tension and muscular strength may also be due to this.

It is interesting to note that this male climacteric or 'menopause' appears in men at or shortly after the 'retiral phase'. That is, just as women are 'retiring' generally speaking from the role of mother, they develop hormonal changes, and just as men are retiring from the working man/breadwinner role, they too develop hormonal changes. This could be taken as an example of the close connexion between the internal 'nature' of man and woman and his or her external environment. It could also be looked at the other way round, that the pattern of social changes is caused by the hormonal phase change. Whichever came first, the results are similar in the need for social and emotional readjustment of the man and the woman.

The fact that the gap between the female menopause and the male climacteric in a given couple may be fifteen years or more should, in theory, allow each sex sufficient time to readjust to new roles, new goals and new needs. Unfortunately, the individual variation in the effects of menopause and climacteric as well as the variation in time gap may make interpersonal stability less easy to achieve. This could mean, within marriage, that sexual difficulties arising from the altered hormonal states may never be properly resolved, despite the help (if it is sought) of doctor, marriage guidance counsellor and psychiatrist. Nevertheless, it is obviously worth seeking professional help if relationships do deteriorate. Both being able to talk about problems to an unprejudiced hearer, and being given insight into the mutual changes in the physical and psychological states of each partner, will at least offer a better chance of resolution if resolution is possible.

Single men no less than married men undergo the changes of the climacteric we have described. They, too, have to adjust to the changes of hormonal state which may coincide with their retirement. Unless they live as hermits (and even then they may still have sexual needs and sexual outlet), they also find interpersonal relationships with the opposite or their own sex are affected both in emotional and sexual aspects. Unfortunately they have no obvious source of help or guidance like the marriage guidance council, although doctors and psychiatrists are often willing to listen and advise, and prescribe appropriately.

When the sex hormones were first discovered, it was thought that here at last was the medieval 'elixir of life'. Enthusiasts conjectured that giving female hormones to older females and male hormones to older males would ward off senescence and true ageing. In the famous monkey-gland experiments, testicles of the chimpanzee were grafted into old men in the hope and belief that rejuvenation would devolve. Today we understand from our knowledge of immune mechanisms that such grafts would be rejected as 'foreign to self' by the recipient body. Moreover, it is clear that although sex hormones in the hormone-deficient can produce improvement in mental and physical wellbeing and, in appropriate cases, return or maintenance of sexual function, there is no question of the hormones extending the furthest limits of the human life span.

The reports of treatment with testosterone (by sublingual pellets or intramuscular injection, and more recently with testosterone implants) in patients suffering from the 'male climacteric' or evidence of testicular defect in ageing, are sometimes very disappointing. They show that the increase in general wellbeing (with loss of apathy and depression and subsequent gain in weight and strength) outweighs the improvement in sexual function and return of sexual tensions. Whether this is because the dosage of testosterone is still too low in its present form, or whether it is because of the overall hardening of the arteries, may well be determined as research in this field continues. Nevertheless a number of workers have published encouraging results in the treatment of impotence in older males who were deficient in testosterone. Either testosterone implants or the newer fluoxymesterone by mouth was used and this kind of therapy is always considered in appropriate cases. As we shall see in the next chapter, however, the problem of impotence is more likely to be a predominantly psychological one than a physical one.

Doctors are aware of a flaw in the prescription of testosterone in older males. The incidence of unsuspected cancer of the prostate gland, at the base of the bladder, is much commoner after the age of seventy. The cancer grows well in the presence of testosterone, being what is called 'a hormone-dependent growth'. In fact, the female hormone, stilboestrol, is given to retard cancer of the prostate. Thus, patients about to embark on testosterone therapy for any reason must have a careful physical and chemical examination to exclude the presence of any prostrate cancer, and should not be given any testosterone if it is present or suspected.

There are similar flaws in the continued administration

of oestrogens in women. Cancer of the breast in women is often 'hormone-dependent' and the giving of oestrogens will maintain or worsen a malignant breast growth, once it is present. The same, as we have noted, holds true for cancer of the womb. Women on hormones during and after the menopause must have regular check-up examinations of breasts and womb by their family doctor or at their local cancer screening clinic. Another medical disadvantage of 'preventing the menopause' by oestrogen hormones is that two other gynaecological illnesses may be encouraged – neither of them malignant or fatal but both troublesome and normally 'burned out' at the menopause. (These are endo-metriosis and the benign myomas.)

For those who are unhappy about taking hormones by mouth, the use of local stilboestrol or other oestrogenic cream is recommended for the vaginal mucosa. The cream is not absorbed into the bloodstream and no systemic hormone effects are ever noted. Such a cream will not therefore sup-press the symptoms and general signs of the menopause, which we have already discussed.

Sometimes both male and female older patients show evidence of non-specific thinning of muscles and bones which is related to a 'negative nitrogen balance'. This can partly be overcome by encouraging an increased intake of good protein foods like meat, chicken, eggs and fish – but these are more expensive than the starch and sugar foods favoured by fixed-income groups like pensioners. Doctors therefore may prescribe 'anabolic' or protein-building hormones by mouth or by injection. These have no direct effect on sexual function but sexual performance may be improved with the improvement in general health.

Need there be a Pause?

There is a well-known neurologist of the Scottish school whose lectures on diseases of the nervous system are always popular and well attended by the medical students. The reason for the undergraduate doctors' unusual affection for the spoken word lies in the neurologist's approach to his speciality and in the appeal of his presentation of illnesses of the spinal, cranial and other nerve systems. One of his favourite ploys is to demonstrate the essence of an illness by plotting the patient's history and progress of symptoms as a graph. Certain graph patterns give a strong clue to the ultimate diagnosis.

Most people think of the sexual life graph – age plotted against sexual outlet – as a straight line. The line rises sharply from base to high levels at puberty and young adulthood. From this zenith, another straight line descends gradually in the thirties and forties, and then falls away steeply to reach baseline again by the fifties. This popular idea of the sexual life graph is partly based on the changing hormonal state of males and females which we have already discussed. The 'straight line' fall to base at the fifties is more of a myth than a reality. Instead there may be a levelling out at the menopause of the 'straight line' as partners readjust to middle age and menopausal changes. Then the line can begin to climb again, producing a 'reversed plateau'.

Moreover, in the case of the female, we have seen that oestrogen deficiency with its emotional and physical disadvantages can be overcome with hormonal therapy. When the line begins to fall again for the male in the late sixties, hormonal therapy may or may not reverse the graph. If it does reverse it, there is another inverted plateau and the line drops later to base level when other factors – poor or failing health, loss of sex partner, arteriosclerotic changes

– terminate sex function though not necessarily sex interest.

The question, 'need there be a pause?' can be answered in several ways. If there are marked menopausal symptoms requiring hormone therapy and sexual readjustment, then the answer is, temporarily, yes. If the symptoms are minimal and the partners can continue mutual physical interest and enjoyment, the answer is, emphatically, no. If the additive effects of middle age call for a phase of personal reassessment and interpersonal readjustment, the answer may be either temporarily yes, or permanently no – that is a cessation instead of a pause. In other words, the important consideration is, in the individual case or for the individual couple, why is there a pause and can it be shortened or overcome by appropriate help in terms of advice and medical therapy? It is often pointed out that, in marriage, a couple can have an apparently successful married life with limited sexual relationships, so the further question may be asked, 'is it all that important to determine, at middle age, a cause and a solution for diminished or absent sexual intercourse?' The answer to this lies in the importance which each partner gives to his or her sexual tension and outlet, and the significant role their mutual sexual outlet plays in the dynamics of their married life.

3 | The Changing Mind

Fear of Failure

Among the fears of older people, fear of loneliness and fear of death are well-known. For voluntary and professional workers in the field of human ageing, combating the lonely state – which leads to mental apathy, depression and physical neglect – is a major activity. Luncheon and over-sixties clubs, guild and church meetings, charity functions and whist drives, home visitors, day centres and day hospitals, golf and bowling groups, night school and day classes – all these and more are suitable antidotes to loneliness, boredom and gloomy introspection, enhancing the common anxieties that the future may bring economic want, increasing disability and ill-health. The fear of death, which has been with us all to a greater or lesser degree from the onset of maturity, is likely also at this time to become more pressing, though it is often assuaged by material and spiritual comforts, the rewards of work well done, of parenthood and grandparenthood, and by the pleasure of memory.

Such fears are universally admitted, and are not considered shameful or to require suppression. An equally common and important fear among older men, however, that is supposedly shaming and that cannot be publicly acknowledged, is the fear of impotence. Under differing circumstances, older members of the population in this country may worry over a falling off of sexual function but may not approach their doctors for fear of ridicule or reproof – 'really, worrying at your age!' Other circumstances that may lead to inquiry about possible impotence are familiar to doctors practising genito-urinary surgery and to family doctors. In the former case, the older male may be suffering from signs of an enlarged prostate gland – frequency at night and by day, poor stream, slow commencement of stream – so that a prostatectomy for removal of the gland is recommended. If the man is still enjoying an active sexual life, he may surmise from 'hearsay' that this will be brought to an end by the operation, and he will ask the surgeon for his opinion on this matter. The answer is not an easy one. The influence of the mind is so great that merely anticipating that he will be impotent may be sufficient to produce that result. However, the surgeon can usually reassure the patient that the operation is not likely to affect erection or ability to achieve orgasm, or the ejaculatory mechanism for that matter.

Fear of impotency may arise when the family doctor or specialist recommends a male patient for an operation in the area of the genitals. On the other hand, the need for such an operation, or the fact of such an operation having been performed, may be used as a 'laudable excuse' for discontinuing unwanted or unsatisfactory sexual relations. Problems 'down below', to use the vernacular, can always be used as reasons for withdrawing from sexual activity.

Another example where fear of impotence has been noted concerns the older man marrying a young or younger woman. Both the bachelor and the man who is remarrying may anticipate failure in the sexual role and seek medical advice, before the wedding day. As well as seeking reassurance on his physical condition, the prospective bridegroom may ask for a suitable stimulant as an insurance against failure. Of course impotence in other situations, real or anticipated, may encourage the man to buy and try advertised aphrodisiacs or ask his doctor for a prescription. The doctor, on the other hand, is well aware that the female body, clothed or naked, is the strongest aphrodisiac for the heterosexual male. He is therefore not unreasonably doubtful about the value or success of 'synthetic' stimulants in the impotent man. (The younger man who comes to the doctor complaining of 'impotence' and asking for a prescription may in fact be referring to premature ejaculation. This particular form of sexual malfunction is so common as to be considered 'normal'. Such factors as undue sensitivity of the tip of the penis, or the slower arousal of the woman in contrast to the rapid excitation of the man, make premature emission of semen more likely. The latter is particularly common as a factor in the early months or years of a sexual relationship, and appears to be commoner in sexual partners with a higher intelligence quotient and a better economic status.)

Before considering this matter further, let us look at the physiological mechanisms underlying the processes of male potency. Overlording the hormones and nerves which control the process of erection and ultimate ejaculation, the cerebral cortex of the brain can alter or modify the reaction. Stimulating or inhibiting, it can function in a different manner in the same person on different occasions. The sex organs involved are the penis, the prostate gland, and the seminal vesicles. The testicles are bystanders, apart from their important production of testosterone hormone. On receipt of the 'erotic message' from the brain – following visual, auditory, olfactory or other sexual stimuli – the nerves from the lower part of the spinal cord send out their own messages to the 'nervi erigentes' which allow the spongy tissue of the penis to open and fill up with blood. The organ passes from its flabby drooping state to its rigid erect state, at an angle slightly above the horizontal. This first stage in potency having been reached, further messages will be issued from the brain or other parts (fingers, lips, general body contact) and from local friction of the sensitive end of the penis. These reach the prostate and seminal vesicles which express their fluid and semen into the back of the urethra (the outlet of the penis). Still further messages motivate the muscles at the base of the penis, which contract and expel the ejaculate in a rhythmic movement. This ejaculation represents the second part of male potency.

Thus impotence can mean failure of erection, failure of ejaculation or failure of both. Any factor which interrupts the nerves supplying the penis will prevent erection. Any factor interrupting the nerves to the prostate and seminal vesicles, and to the muscles at the base of the penis, will prevent ejaculation. In the under-fifties, psychological factors are the commonest cause; that is, poor erotic responsiveness or psychological immaturity, the fear of failure or other mental barriers. Organic (non-psychological) factors can be important too, and should not be overlooked as in the following example. A pleasant young man of thirty-five, married, with two children, was attending a medical outpatient department. One day his wife came with him and while he was undressing for examination in another room, she quietly asked the doctor why her husband had lost 'his nature'. Further questioning revealed that he had difficulty in erection and (even more) in ejaculation although he was normally excited by erotic stimuli. This had started fairly soon after attending the outpatient clinic for the first time. The doctor considered some sort of related psychological explanation. However, when he examined the patient and began to take his blood pressure which had been fairly high before treatment, he recalled the obvious medical point. The young man was having pills to lower high blood pressure. The pills sometimes interfere with the sympathetic and para-sympathetic nerves from the lower part of the spinal cord – the nerves of male potency.

This patient was an example of drug-induced impotence with retention of sexual desire (libido). Drugs may also depress sexual tension with reduction or loss of libido.

For example, a man of twenty-eight was referred to a medical outpatients because of recurring epileptic fits. When interviewed, he told the doctor that he had had fits occasionally since his teens for which he had taken phenobarbitone prescribed by his family doctor. He had never taken much interest in girls although he mixed with a contemporary male crowd who enjoyed sexual flirtation and adventure. Recently he had taken up with a girl as part of a 'foursome' and was surprised when she complained at his lack of amorous advances. With fair insight, he wondered if his regular tablets were interfering with his sexual desires, and therefore stopped taking them. He admitted that his sexual interest and need for sexual outlet were now quite strong but, unfortunately, his fits, which had been suppressed by the phenobarbitone, were back in force. The 'remedy' was to replace the phenobarbitone with a different anti-convulsant which did not interfere with his libido but suppressed his fits. Both the patient and, presumably, his girlfriend were grateful.

Sedatives, hypnotics and tranquillizing drugs are commonly prescribed in the older age groups where anxiety, insomnia and neurosis require treatment. These drugs must always be considered as a possible factor when patients complain of loss of libido or impotence. We noted in the last chapter that female hormones, like stilboestrol, may be given in the treatment of prostatic cancer and this, as one might expect, would reduce male desire if not potency. Disease or injury involving the lumbo-sacral outflow of the spinal cord nerves can interfere with potency at any age. It may occur with tumours of the lower spinal cord or for example a road or works accident involving the spine. (In the latter case, priapism in which there is persistent penile engorgement and erection may occur.)

Again, as we have noted, failure of testosterone hormone production from immature testicles may result in impotence from boyhood. This can be treated by testosterone implants. Testicular removal (orchidectomy), for any reason, after puberty may reduce sexual tensions although successful sexual intercourse may still be achieved because of the nerve 'reflex' system described above.

One of the important degenerative diseases affecting the over-fifty-fives is arteriosclerosis. This pathological thickening, hardening and narrowing of the arteries can affect the blood supply to brain, heart, muscle and nerves as the years go on. The progress is very variable from one older person to the next, but some people develop personality and intellectual changes from hardening of the cerebral arteries. This condition, known as arteriosclerotic dementia, is phasic but gradually relapsing. A narrowed and fixed outlook, labile emotions, forgetfulness of recent events, introspection and anxiety lead on to more marked intellectual changes and emotional vacuity. Apathy alternating with restlessness, and poor orientation for time and place may follow. This 'senile' picture is the one which is so often equated with 'being old' – it is in fact a brain disease in the older person and is not a characteristic of normal old age.

In arteriosclerotic dementia, there is generally loss of sexual tensions and loss of potency. Alternatively, loss of the cultural and mature inhibitions may lead to unexpected or anti-social sexual activities.

Another illness in which impotence may appear with retention of libido is the condition of sugar diabetes – more properly called diabetes mellitus. Considering the number of known and latent diabetic men in the general population, this is a relatively unusual side-effect. It may be due to the changes in the small blood vessels that supply the nervi erigentes and other 'sexual' nerves (diabetic arteriopathy), or it may be due to the basic biochemical disturbance of diabetes mellitus interfering with the nourishment of the 'sexual' nerves.

Hope of Success

If impotence in older men is to be overcome, then a decision must be made by the appropriate authority – physician, psychiatrist, family doctor for example – as to the relative roles of the organic or physical factors, and the mental or psychological factors in each individual case. There is no simple rule of thumb which will lead to a quick answer in any case of male impotence. The affected man may look for short cuts to an answer, such as using tablets, creams or appliances that are offered to him by helpful advertisers or well-meaning lay persons. Discreet and overt advertisements for products that are said to be helpful in premature ejaculation or sexual fatigue are not as abundant in this country's literature and hoardings as they are abroad.

Since there are few physical complaints which do not also have a psychological component or overtone, it is not surprising that impotence may be a difficult problem to treat in the individual case. To take the organic condition of testosterone deficiency as an example, there is no simple test for this as there is in the case of female oestrogen deficiency. In the woman, as we noted, microscopic examination of a smear taken from the neck of the womb, in a consulting-room examination that is pain-free and quick, will readily reveal whether she is mildly, moderately or severely short of oestrogen. Such a straightforward cell test is not available in men. The biochemical test in men involves collecting a twenty-four hour sample of the urine in the first place. Next, in the biochemical laboratory special chemical techniques are used to measure the substances known as 17-oxosteroids in the urine sample. The result gives an estimate of the total male hormone production, not just from the testicles but also from the two adrenal glands in the loin. The laboratory figure of ten to twenty-five mgm in twenty-four hours is the accepted range in the adult male, and this figure falls below ten mgm in the seventh decade in the majority of male patients studied.

An actual estimate of the testosterone production in twenty-four hours can be made and the figure is around eighteen mgm in young healthy adults. This figure rises with exercise, suggesting that the 'keep fit' propagandists may have a point in their 'healthier life' programmes. Middle-aged or older men who complain of loss of sexual desire or of impotence in the act, and who have a very low oxosteroid excretion in twenty-four hours (or a low actual testosterone output), can be given a trial of hormones. They are given either a testosterone implant or fluoxymesterone by mouth, in doses which raise the 17-oxosteroid excretion to near normal levels. Clinical reports vary as to the improvement in libido and sex function in hormone-deficient males so treated. In some, the treatment seems to be most beneficial, and in others there is little or no change. In some, only trans-ient improvement is seen, suggesting a psychological effect. Some doctors have added small quantities of female hor-mone to the male hormone. This male-female hormone treatment is said to be more true to nature and possibly more successful.

Since the anterior pituitary gland in the brain influences the testicles to produce testosterone, it has been suggested that giving gonadotrophins might help patients with im-potence. (Gonadotrophins have been used in primary fail-ure of the pituitary in young women, to stimulate the ovaries to produce ova. The influence on libido or orgasm has not been reported.) This is not as likely to be successful as the giving of fluoxymesterone or testosterone implants.

In the other organic causes of impotence – drug therapy, injury, tissue injury and disease – treatment of the cause where possible, should improve the picture and give the patient so treated 'hope of success'. The psychological effect of having failed, however, calls for reassurance by the counsellor or doctor, for even after a mild illness in an older man – influenza or bronchitis – the man may find some difficulty in maintenance of an erection, or premature ejaculation may occur. This in turn may lead to loss of sexual confidence, especially if there is poor understanding from his female partner. Persistence of a painful illness, for example rheumatoid arthritis or post-herpetic neuralgia, may psychologically dampen libido and encourage permanent impotence.

We have already noted the importance of reassuring men undergoing prostate operations or other operations in the genital region. Here, too, initial post-operative 'failure' of sexual connexion may depress libido and result in psychologically determined impotence. The effects of mental illness are also important and I shall discuss this shortly. In the older male patient, who is otherwise mentally healthy and physically fit, and whose 17-oxosteroids are not especially deficient, the treatment of impotence will involve psychotherapy which enlists not only the patient's own help but also that of his female partner.

The occurrence of morning erections (waking with the penis engorged and erect) is a normal phenomenon in healthy adults and may continue well into old age. It is sometimes thought that morning erections – proving that the hormone and nerve supply to the penis is intact – imply that the man must be potent for the sexual situation. This is not necessarily so. For example, a man aged fifty-eight, an ex-labourer, was attending an outpatient clinic for follow-up after a minor left-sided 'stroke'. Recovery was excellent but the patient complained of impotence with his wife who was ten years younger. On inquiry, he stated he was still having morning erections but, when he and his wife tried to take advantage of this he was unable to ejaculate or have orgasm.

Notwithstanding this example, where the impotence is

psychological the presence of morning erections at least indicates that function can occur and puts therapy on a surer basis. The next step is to determine whether the female partner – wife or regular mate – is an intrinsic reason for the loss of potency. A woman aged forty-two, previously happily married, attended the medical outpatients complaining of marked weight gain, loss of scalp hair, constipation and feeling the cold even in warm rooms. She was slow in her responses and, telling her story, revealed that both she and her husband were considering divorce. Apparently she had begun to lose her libido but even before this was complete her husband had become impotent with her. However, he had managed sexual relations with another woman and felt that 'it was the wife's fault'. The woman was, in fact, suffering from hypothyroidism and responded well over the next few months to oral thyroxine. She lost her excess weight, her scalp hair strengthened, her bowel function improved and her entire appearance went from one of 'rapid ageing' to one of normal forties. On a routine visit for follow-up, she stated that her husband was now 'a man again' with her, that is, that sexual intercourse was satisfactory. Her libido had returned and his impotence had been based on revulsion to his wife's previous disease-altered appearance.

Unfortunately, not every case has such a happy ending. In particular, where husbands have depended on the physical facial and bodily attractiveness of their wives to stimulate erotic arousal, facial and body changes as a result of operation, injury or hormonal change may result in impotence in the marriage bed or bedroom.

Different coital positions can be recommended which either allow an erection to be held for longer periods or stimulate erection or ejaculation. This may meet with some opposition from either or both partners. The reasons for this antagonism are considered in the next section.

Change of Approach

The factors which influence a choice of sexual partner are both individual and universal. Universal factors include the physical and hormonal make-up of men and women which generally predisposes them to choose partners from the opposite sex and from the species homo sapiens. Individual factors are numerous and, in a given case, will be determined both by conscious recognition of pleasing aspects of the chosen partner, and by unconscious conditioned stimuli which stem from childhood and pre-maturity. We shall be discussing the influence of Sigmund Freud in a later chapter, but few laymen are unaware of the stress which Freud laid on childhood experiences in predetermining many aspects of our sexual (and everyday) behaviour in adult life. Mothers, encouraged by child guidance manuals quoting psychoanalytic predictions, no longer restrain their childrens' behaviour at home or in company, and no longer give laxatives to clear out the bowels while chastising the child who is not yet toilet trained, for the dangers of repression and frustration producing neuroses and sexual and behavioural instability are well understood in the nurseries of today.

The factors which stimulate a rise in the level of sexual tension and a desire for sexual outlet are also both individual and universal. For the male sex as a whole, where heterosexual attitudes predominate, any object which is inherently feminine – like skirts, dresses, lingerie, high-heeled shoes, handbags – or any object which is feminine by association – like perfume, make-up, hair pieces – or any object which is feminine by observation – such as pin-up studies, girlie calendars, film and television females – can all produce arousal of various degrees. In the individual male, in addition to these general objects of arousal there are conditioned responses, so that one man may be aroused only by the sight of his wife's nakedness, a second man may be aroused only by the sight of his wife partially unclothed, and a third man may be aroused merely by the sight of his wife's nightwear hanging in the cupboard. Or, for example, one man may be aroused by any woman with blonde hair and blue eyes, another man be aroused by any woman who resembles the 'sex bomb' image of the day, and yet another man may be roused only when his partner wears shiny plastic garments.

For the female sex as a whole, where heterosexual attitudes predominate, the factors which raise the level of sexual tension are much more individual, and based on conditioning of a personal kind, than in the male. They are not universally aroused by objects which are inherently male or·male by association or male by observation. They may still be aroused on an individual basis by observation of love play on films or television, by reading erotic chapters in novels, by seeing the partner naked or partially unclothed, by particular colour of hair and eyes, by hairiness or smooth skin, and by very individual associations like smells, a piece of music and a particular physical contact.

We suggested in the last section that the adoption of different positions in sexual intercourse is worth considering in some cases of male impotence. The factors which lead a couple to use a particular position for sexual intercourse are multiple. They include such points as the time and place of opportunity, the breadth of sexual knowledge, the tradition and customs of the social group to which the couple belong, the length of sexual experience, the health of the partners, the presence or absence of clothing and the desire for an unfamiliar approach to a familiar pleasure.

With reference to the tradition and customs of the social group to which the couple belong, such traditions tend to influence the couple to believe that only certain positions of intercourse are 'normal'. Experimenting or even reading about other positions for the sexual act provokes guilt feelings which either or both partners may ignore or not. Adding guilt to the impotence situation may only aggravate that situation. Reassurance by doctor or counsellor that a 'normal' position for intercourse is in fact any position that is comfortable, functional and mutually satisfying, may help to overcome the experimenting couple's guilt and self-censure.

While some couples are prepared to experiment when the male partner has difficulty in erection (or in holding an erection to ejaculation), other couples are inhibited by the conditioning factors noted above and need guidance and re-assurance if a change of sexual approach is contemplated. Provided the hormonal, nerve and blood supply of the sexual organ is intact, the fact that the man is middle-aged or older does not preclude a trial of new coital positions. Apathetic or unimaginative couples or partners may find such a change of approach 'too much bother' so that the sexual relationship breaks down.

Assuming the most popular position for sexual intercourse is that of the man lying on top of the woman, we can then consider variations which might help in the impotence situation. The first possibility is that the woman can lie on top of the man. Such a position allows the insertion and firmer vaginal holding of even a partially erect penis. (The method has been used successfully by paraplegics who wished to inseminate their wives, despite their own loss of feeling and movement below the waist from their illness.) The female partner provides most of the initial rhythmic movements and may be able to promote ejaculation as well as erection. The next possibility is the use of a side-to-side approach. Either the man faces the woman, each lying on the side, or the man approaches the woman from the rear for vaginal entrance, each lying on the side. If the woman lies first slightly higher, then slightly lower than the man, compression of the penis backwards can help to promote and maintain erection or proceed to ejaculation.

Raising the level of the vaginal entrance in the position of woman underneath the man, for example by a foam pad or a cushion, again tends to compress the penis backwards as it enters the orifice. Sometimes the adoption of a sitting position with the man behind the woman for rear vaginal entrance promotes a similar result. Yet another possibility is for the woman to draw up her knees before parting the legs, instead of having the legs extended, in the woman under the man position. Whatever new approach is used, success is unlikely to be immediate, and sympathetic consideration of the partners for each other needs to be present and maintained.

In addition to a change in approach, the doctor or counsellor can advise the partners on the use of external erotic stimuli, provided it is known to which objects and subjects the impotent male has been sexually conditioned in the past. The ploy of varying the room or place within the room, of adding dim light and familiar 'mood' background music, of the female partner wearing sexually stimulating bedwear, has been known to generations of 'seducers' and there is no reason to suppose that such environmental stimulating factors cannot be helpful in male impotence. The nude oil painting that is traditionally said to adorn the Frenchman's bedroom would be just as valuable in the Englishman's bedroom, even if it is not Renoir's 'Gabrielle'.

In an earlier part of this chapter, I noted that an impotent man might seek a short cut to his problem by sending for tablets or creams which are advertised as remedies for 'male sexual problems'. Such tablets may contain harmless small quantities of vitamins, perhaps with the addition of iron, and perhaps a dye which impressively changes the colour of the urine but has no other pharmacological effect. Other tablets may contain small doses of amphetamine or chemically similar brain stimulant which are designed to 'give the sufferer a mental lift'. More dangerous drugs which are said to be sex stimulants but which in fact chemically irritate the bladder base and the urethra are obtained illegally by some remedy seekers. The most lethal of these drugs is cantharides, which is poisonous even in small doses and is not an aphrodisiac at all.

Most cultures place an aphrodisiac quality on at least one food. Whether it is oysters or caviare, for example, doctors know that the effects of the food are not physical but based on the psychological factor of suggestion. Alcohol in moderate doses is known to reduce social inhibitions and may encourage erotic thoughts in some individuals. However, even if it increases the mental desire, it reduces the physical performance and cannot be recommended to the impotent man.

The fact that sedatives and tranquillizers can lower sexual tension was noted earlier. However, somewhat paradoxically, tranquillizers have proved helpful in some cases of impotence where anxiety and tension have been brought under control by their use. There is one drug firm that produces a product containing an extract of South American tree bark, a tiny dose of strychnine, a stimulant and a sedative and some male hormone all compounded in one tablet. This example of polypharmacy is presumably designed to cover all the avenues of drug treatment in this problem.

Whatever drug therapy is used in the treatment of impotence, it is not likely to succeed fully without the addition of reassurance and psychotherapy. Moreover, drugs should be used only under strict medical supervision.

Sex and the Longer Life

Women, Equality and Frigidity

Improved opportunities for education, commercial and industrial training, and career work have raised the status of women in the community, but the role of the woman in the sexual sphere is still far from emancipated. In our culture, the principle that man is the dominant partner in a sexual relationship is still strongly entrenched. Feminine enjoyment of sex play is admitted but the idea of a strong female sexual appetite is played down or denied. That women can perform as equal sex partners with men, and not just simply be passive playthings, is a suggestion that may not go down too well even with scientific or medical men. Among the latter, a patriarchal attitude to sexual relations is all too common especially in the older generations. We have observed in the chapter on the female menopause that some gynaecologists are but little perturbed at the diminution or loss of sexual tension in that phase.

The attitude of male dominance is simply an extension of the moral and legal outlook of earlier centuries and of the Judaic and Christian and Far Eastern cultures. The role of women in the sex act was generally assumed to be passive, and admission or expression of enjoyment and desire indicated a would-be or an actual harlot. That this attitude is still with us in fair measure was revealed a few years back with the re-publication of John Cleland's classic *Fanny Hill*. The censure of the establishment arose not so much from the descriptive passages on sexual activity – passages which are well paralleled in contemporary novels – but from the obvious delight and gratification that Fanny Hill obtained as an active participant in sexual adventures. There was no similar censure forthcoming when the sexual activities of Henry Miller were described in the re-published *Tropic of Capricorn*.

In women as in men the range of sexual tension levels and

the need for sexual outlets vary widely, from very great to very little, over the general population. Moreover, it appears that self-awareness and self-understanding of sexual tensions and sexual outlets is slower to mature in the female, even though the age of onset of the average female puberty (menstruation, development of breasts, growth of pubic and axillary hair) may be at the same time or earlier than average male puberty (changes of voice, growth of pubic and axillary hair, ability for erection and ejaculation). Certainly the male has no difficulty in recognizing the focal point of his sexuality in the urge to penetrate the female and ejaculate his semen. Orgasm – the highest level of sexual tension in the excitement of the sex act – is soon recognized by the male. The female, however, slower to arousal and more easily distracted in sexual intercourse, may never achieve the highest level of tension and relief in an orgasmic experience, even though she may be well satisfied with the sex play and subsequent sexual intercourse.

Since a woman does not have to achieve erection of a phallic organ in order to participate in sexual intercourse, it is usual to designate loss or lack of libido, and female sexual dissatisfaction, by the term 'frigidity', and not to use the term 'impotence'. While I appreciate the technical differences that might lead to a different nomenclature for a similar problem, it is salutary to remember that impotence means that an unresponding male has simply (to transliterate) lost his power, while the corresponding female frigidity means that the female is chillingly stiff. These terms are a further indication of the male-proposed role that normally woman should be warmingly relaxed and that normally man should be sexually powerful.

The term 'frigidity' is itself often poorly defined, being applied to one woman, for example, who has no desire for sexual intercourse; to another woman who has some sexual tension, seeking outlet in coitus but infrequently; to a third woman who has regular coitus but fails to achieve orgasm; or to yet another who acquiesces in coitus but objects to being touched by the hands of her sexual partner. In other words, the word is used to connote the gap between the 'expected' level of sexual tension and frequency and enjoyment of sexual outlet, and the actual individual level and frequency and enjoyment. It may be used as a simple statement of 'fact', or as a verbal whiplash; as a call for help from either the frigid woman or her disappointed spouse, or from both.

As we noted in the case of the male that impotence in the form of premature ejaculation is common in the earlier years of married life, so it is not unusual for the female to have lower levels of sexual desire in the first months of marriage, compared with her spouse. This is not to deny the presence of sexual tensions in the healthy young female, but these may be masked by the initial persistence of her previous social training, or lack of training, on sexual matters. The attitudes, spoken and unspoken, of her parents and teachers on sexual matters and towards the sexual organs and sexual intimacy, are of great influence. If mother passes on to daughter an attitude of 'men are beasts, they need sex and we don't', or 'give the man sex to keep him happy but don't expect to enjoy it', or 'sex is disgusting but necessary to have children', or 'it isn't ladylike to be seen naked even in marriage' – such sex-debasing and sex-debunking information puts the inexperienced newly-married female at a great disadvantage. If sexual intercourse then proves as unappetizing or unpleasurable as was 'expected', permanent disenchantment with coitus (and with man from this aspect) may result. Not surprisingly, the female may pass on her feelings and experience in turn to the next generation of womanhood.

While freer discussion of sexual matters abounds in public places (the mass entertainment media), good educational facilities in the anatomy, physiology and hygiene of sex and the psychological aspects of sexual relationships are not universally available to the senior schoolchildren and adolescents of the United Kingdom. Moreover, the influence of the establishment attitude towards sexuality in women is still great in the home, in the school and in the places of religion. To this – the passive role of woman in sex – is added the romantic façade, which implies that she can enjoy marriage emotionally in terms of 'happily-ever-aftering' but not in 'orgasm-ever-aftering'. While, as I have stated in an earlier chapter, I do not underrate romance in human relationships, it is no substitute for realistic adjustment of the marriage partners in their day-to-day physical, mental and emotional meeting points.

In the case of the male in older life, we have seen that both organic and psychological factors in greater or lesser degree influence the individual case of impotence. Let us look at the organic factors in the female first. The effects of drug treatment for illness are just as likely to be depressive sexually in women as they are in men. The phenothiazine tranquillizers are widely used for anxiety states and neurosis. They are also therapeutic for mental disturbances in physical illness, like insomnia and irritability. These drugs can reduce sexual desire and inhibit sexual outlet in many women treated with them. (Paradoxically, however, the calming effect of these drugs can be used in treating psychological frigidity.) The barbiturates, used as sleep-inducers or as anti-epileptic pills, also may interfere with libido in susceptible women. Drugs used in the treatment of medical illnesses, like the sympatholytic drugs for high blood pressure, may reduce sexual reactiveness in the female as well as in the male. Giving female hormones, like stilboestrol, to the male (as mentioned in the treatment for cancer of the prostate), will feminize the man physically and reduce his sexual tensions and need of outlet. The female

93

given male sex hormones, like testosterone (for the treatment of some cancers of the breast), may well show an increase of libido, with desire for more frequent coitus or other form of sexual outlet. Whether the rise in sexual tension is due to augmentation of the libidinizing effect of her own male hormones from the adrenal glands, or whether it is because the sexually sensitive clitoris enlarges considerably, or whether – more likely – it is a combination of the two, this male hormone 'side-effect' in women is well documented.

As with any medical or surgical illness in older men, disease and ill-health in older women is likely to reduce sexual tensions and the need for outlet. Again, ill-health may be used as a legitimate excuse to terminate unsatisfactory sexual relations, or it may be of such a crippling nature – mentally or physically – as to make ordinary sexual intercourse impossible or biologically inadvisable. If sexual tensions still arise in such disabled women, other modes of outlet may be sought or practised such as masturbation by the sexual partner if there is one, or by the woman herself if she is alone.

Earlier we discussed how men undergoing operation for an enlarged prostate gland – or, indeed, undergoing any operation in the region of the genital organs – were apprehensive about loss of sexual potency and loss of libido. In general, it was stated, the surgeon could reassure the man undergoing the operation that his potency and libido were unlikely to be altered. Nevertheless, some men did report impotence post-operatively; but it was felt this was largely a psychological phenomenon which could be overcome, patient and wife willing.

In the case of the female, removal of the womb (hysterectomy) with or without the ovaries, or removal of the ovaries, may invite the same question – 'will this put an end to sexual feeling and desire and enjoyment of intercourse?'

The same answer the surgeon gave the man holds good for the woman. In general, removal of the womb should have no physical effect on sexual tension or the enjoyment of intercourse. In the case of the ovaries – an 'artificial menopause' – we have discussed the effects in an earlier chapter, and how the use of female sex hormones can overcome the effects of the operation on the genital tract and on the psyche. So here again the woman can be reassured. Despite these facts and the rationality of reassurance, the mechanistic or superstitious view that a woman's sexuality lies deep in the womb may prevail in the woman of lower social level or lower intelligence. I recall that one of the characters in James Jones's powerful novel, *From Here to Eternity*, was a woman who castigated her husband for giving her a disease which necessitated the removal of her womb, and the loss of her 'femininity'.

The psychological aspects of frigidity may overlay organic disease or exist as an entity on their own. We have already considered how parental or other authoritarian teaching or implied assertion may denigrate sex as unwholesome, unclean, burdensome and – except as a direct means to procreation – undesirable. Difficult sexual adjustment early in marriage may create interpersonal tensions that persist as the children grow up and the partners mature materially and socially. Thus, the menopause, or the woman returning to a career or taking up, say, charitable work as the children go to school or leave the family unit – all these and other physical or social changes may be used as a lever to throw off uncomfortable, uncomforting, uninviting sexual relations. Alternatively the socio-physical changes of middle age may bring a reappraisal of the marriage partnership so that the female, disenchanted, and with new social opportunities, takes up a relationship (temporary or permanent) with a 'new' man. As a result she may be frigid with her 'old' partner.

As we shall see in the next part of this chapter, frigidity may be part of a mental illness of the psychiatric type and may be considered as psychological if the mental sickness goes unrecognized.

Before going on to summarize the patterns of treatment in the above situations, I should consider the type of frigidity in which the woman has sexual tension and the need for sexual outlet, but in whom the usual form of outlet – sexual intercourse – seldom or never produces the highest levels of sexual tension and the relief from these known as orgasm. The interest and importance of female orgasm in sexual relations appears to be a function of the twentieth-century 'discovery' that women can actually have pleasure in the sex act equivalent to the male intromission and ejaculation.

If we consider the physiology of the female sexual parts during sexual intercourse we might discover why some women never reach orgasm. (The percentage of married women who do achieve orgasm does in fact rise with the number of years married, so that many older women – two thirds or more of a given population – enjoy coitus to its maximum even though its frequency is relatively less.) On erotic arousal – either by the stimulus of the situation such as bed, warmth, body contact in nakedness, or by stimulation through kissing or psychological stimulus – the internal lining of the vagina becomes engorged (like the penis) and moist. Next, the clitoris (organ equivalent to, but much smaller than, the penis) which stands just above the entrance to the vagina, receives the same messages from the brain via the spinal cord nerves as did the vagina. Like the penis, it also becomes engorged and this distension increases with psychical excitement and tactile stimulation. The same brain messages come through the spinal cord higher up, producing erection of the nipples. Internally, the vaginal muscles distend the walls to open wider and the lips of the entrance pout apart. This allows entry of the distended penis, which is then held by contraction of the proximal vaginal portion. Easier entrance takes place if Bartholini's glands lubricate the inner vaginal lips. Both in the male and female partner, there are the usual general effects of rapid breathing, increased heart rate and slight rise in blood pressure. Sooner or later, the male ejaculates as he comes to orgasm. The female may not reach orgasm, however, but if she does, after further clitoral stimulation the vaginal muscles contract rhythmically and the womb above may contract also. While the male detumescence prevents further erections for some time, further rhythmical contractions of the vagina are quite possible, so that the female may have more than one orgasm in the sexual act. Let me stress again that many women enjoy sex play and sexual intercourse without necessarily reaching orgasm. Sexual tensions arising at any age, seeking a sexual outlet, can be assuaged by minor or major sexual contact. It is obvious that orgasm in the woman is not needed to ensure conception after sexual intercourse, for the emission of semen at a barely penetrated vaginal entrance has often led to an unexpected pregnancy. The question may be posed as to whether it is worth bothering if some women have orgasm and some do not, as long as sexual happiness is apparent. There are several reasons for answering that orgasm is 'worth bothering about'.

In the first place, if sexual outlet in intercourse gives a woman joy and pleasure, then orgasm will increase that joy and pleasure both physically and mentally. Next, if the woman can sometimes achieve orgasm coincidentally with her male partner, this will increase and deepen their mutual satisfaction in mutual sexual outlet. Thirdly, a woman who can achieve orgasm in other forms of sexual outlet when sexual intercourse is not available to her, is more likely to maintain her sexuality as part of her integral femininity.

Fourthly, the encouragement of women to seek orgasm in sexual outlet is an encouragement to equalize the sexual roles of men and women still further. The sex counsellor's advice is not 'what you've never had, you'll never miss' but rather 'why forego an outstanding feminine experience?'

The outline of the physiology of coitus and orgasm already given leads us to several clues about sexual inadequacy in terms of orgasm. The mental state of the woman is important. She must be in a sexually stimulating environment while additional stimulation from the physical contact of her partner initiates erotic messages to brain and spinal cord. This erotic stimulation should build up effectively to engorge vagina and clitoris. Distractions such as noises, odours, non-erotic thoughts can disturb the nerve messages which produce congestion and erection. The moistening of the vaginal lining is important to lubricate the passage of the penis.

There is no doubt that, once orgasm has been achieved several times in successive acts of coitus, it becomes easier to achieve. For the female who is regularly active sexually through her married years, and who more often than not has orgasm in coitus, there seems to be no upper age limit for orgasm: this assumes good physical and mental health and the maintenance of satisfactory oestrogen levels. On the other hand, since coital frequency for the woman is liable to decrease with age – for the reasons that husbands tend to be several years older than their spouses, that husbands tend to have higher rates of ill-health in middle age, and that husbands die off sooner – her opportunity for orgasm is less and her capacity likely to diminish on that account.

In order to increase libido, and in order to increase clitoral sensitivity, the giving of male sex hormones, like testosterone, has been recommended by doctors in some cases of frigidity. Here again, the support of reassurance and psychotherapy is always necessary. The use of other so-called aphrodisiacs has already been cautioned against in the previous section on male impotence.

For the man, as we have seen, petting, sex play and a variation in the position for intercourse help to produce and maintain his sexual excitement and therefore his erection. The woman, however, being slower in arousal, may need more specific stimulation of the clitoris for some time before she nears orgasm. It has often been found that if she can concentrate on the sexual goal, and if, at the same time, professional help in understanding any psychological difficulties is available, even the woman who has suffered from frigidity for many years can overcome this disability and reach full sexual satisfaction at last. Even where disability precludes the full sexual act, many couples achieve relief of sexual tensions in tender affectionate contact orally or manually, so that this aspect of their married life remains harmonious.

In all the discussion on impotence and on frigidity I have pre-supposed that the affected partner – and, indeed, the opposite sex partner – are keen to maintain sexual relations despite the passage of time in married years and in chronological age. They may well decide, however, that it is 'easier' to opt out and, setting sexual outlets aside, to try and sublimate some of their tensions in other directions. They may be missing some of the richness of the longer life.

Sex and the Longer Life

The ill Mind

I have mentioned several times in the present chapter the importance of mental influences on sexual tensions, needs and outlets. In addition, I have hinted that mental illness by itself can alter sexual patterns and modify the sexual expression of a given individual. This is true in abnormal ageing when there is marked hardening of the brain arteries. In this condition the effects of diminished glucose supply and oxygen supply to the brain – particularly to the intellectual and memory areas of the frontal lobes – results in fluctuating but steadily worsening brain damage. This arteriosclerotic dementia, as it is called, may occur from the late sixties onwards but occasionally occurs in younger age groups.

The clinical features include patchy memory loss, particularly for recent events, poor concentration and inability to grasp ideas and situations. There is apathy, with contrasting restlessness at night, labile emotional reactions or blunting of finer feelings or both, poor judgement and gradual loss of insight. As the illness develops, there is a falling off of sexual tension and desires, and loss of interest towards the female partner as a sexual companion. Sexual outlet may be minimal or absent. At a later stage still, the patient's hygiene suffers and his or her social habits deteriorate. Moreover, the hardened arteries affect the patient's cultural and instinctive sexual inhibitions and there appears to be a reawakening of sexual interest and need for release of sexual tensions. These may be directed towards the opposite sex or show reversion to the auto-erotic stage of sexual development (as outlined by Sigmund Freud). The patient may be virtually impotent, and the absence of coital opportunity may lead to genital exposure, or to interfering sexually with children, or homosexual approaches. Relatively few cases of arteriosclerotic dementia show such

abnormal sexual activity but, if present, it does add to the
already existing difficulties of caring for the patient, attending to the needs of hygiene, and maintaining a sympathetic
attitude in the face of difficult behaviour.

The important point is that abnormal sexuality in ageing
is not a function of chronological age but is a disease that
appears in some old people. Thus older men (and women)
who expose their genitals, or who masturbate in the open,
or who attempt to fondle other people's children are, if
brought before the courts, usually referred for a psychiatric
opinion because they are mentally ill. Psychiatric control
of the abnormal sexual tendencies is usually possible by
means of tranquillizers and psychotropic drugs, but may,
as we have noted, require admission to an appropriate
hospital for further treatment and care, long-term or short-
term. The same pattern is true for 'senile dementia' in
which the breakdown in intellect and personality is rapid
and progressive without the 'remissions' of the arteriosclerotic variety.

Another psychosis (mental illness without obvious insight) that appears in older age groups and interferes with
sexual patterns is depression. Formerly known by the more
expressive name of melancholia, depression is commonly
divided into two types, reactive and endogenous. In the
former, the depressive mood and apathetic state follow on
some stressful event, such as loss of a loved one, but persist
much longer than the expected 'mourning period'. On the
other hand, in the endogenous variety, the change in affect
or emotional state from its normal variability to the persistent depressed state comes slowly 'out of the blue' and is
not obviously related to external circumstances. We have
already noted that depression can arise at the female menopause and this is called involutional depression. Modern
psychiatric treatment is mainly drug-based and includes
the tranquillizers and the newer mood-raising drugs like

imipramine. Electro-shock therapy is still required in some cases. In all forms of depression, there is loss of interest in sexual matters in terms of the need for coitus or other form of sexual outlet. Occasionally patients focus their thoughts on their genital organs as a source of 'sinfulness' and 'uncleanliness' but this is part of the abnormal self-reproach and self-abasement in the psychotic state, and improves to normal attitudes as the depression recedes on treatment. The rarer reverse picture of mania or hypo-mania in which the patient is abnormally active and eupho-ric, with exhausting excited activity, also precludes normal sexual tensions and the desire for outlet.

In the previous parts of this chapter we have seen and discussed the effects of anxiety and neurotic reaction on sexual desire and sexual expression, and pointed out ways and means of overcoming some or most of them. In those cases, it is not so much a question of an 'ill' mind as an 'anxious' one but the same sympathy, care and helpful medical and lay attitudes are needed in any mental upset, and in the further consideration of sexual disturbances of either or both partners.

4 | The Changing Evidence

Freud Reconsidered

Since the beginning of history, sexual needs and sexual behaviour have been topics for discussion, a basis for legal and religious action, a fundament for stories and folklore, an impetus for love, creativeness and war. Not only oral but written traditions are brought down to us from previous oriental and occidental generations. While intellectuals, doctors and psychiatrists, if they belong to the generation before mine, can conjure up such names as Krafft-Ebing or Havelock Ellis, the most universally familiar work on sexual growth and development and the patterns of conscious and unconscious sexual expression is that of the late Professor Sigmund Freud.

My own introduction to the work and original genius of this outstanding Viennese practitioner came through the purchase of a second-hand copy of his *Introductory Lectures on Psychoanalysis*, in a translation by Joan Riviere. This had been published in its first edition in 1922 although my own copy was a later impression. I did not realize at the time I read the book that the logical and well-reasoned contents from the pen of this medically qualified neurologist turned psychoanalyst had initially been ignored and discounted by his contemporaries and later ridiculed and censured by the establishment of his time. Many critics consider Freud's greatest work to be the book *The Interpretation of Dreams*, first published in 1900, but the *Introductory Lectures* are still the most fruitful entrée to Freudian theories. These include his explanation of the structure of the mind, of the growth and organization of sexuality in human beings, of the symbolism and usefulness of dreams, and of the analytical approach to the mental disturbances called neuroses.

Working backwards from his study of neurosis and hysteria and forwards from his understanding of dreams, Freud showed how sexuality does not appear suddenly at puberty but develops slowly through infancy and childhood. This infantile and childhood sexuality is expressed in terms of pleasure and gratification from oral and anal sources, and is eventually moulded to the primacy of the genital areas in sexual gratification. This final development leads neatly onto the reproductive aspect of sexual function after puberty. Freud also illustrated the importance of parent and sibling relationships through the development of erotic complexes, of which the Oedipus complex is justifiably the most famous, and the implication in terms of the family setting of the sexual curiosity of children.

The importance to the future role of sexuality and mental behaviour in the individual attributed to the first six years of life by Freud and other analysts was accepted in Freud's own lifetime. The concept that all aspects of character and personality in adults are moulded in the early years of life has been extended considerably from the original Freudian concept. Sociologists have confirmed this in many ways, such as in John Bowlby's famous study of the effects of parent deprivation in the development of delinquency, in his *Child Care and the Growth of Love*.

The work of Freud, then, confirmed the statement of Wordsworth in the eighteenth century that 'the child is father of the man', although the emphasis on the sexual aspect in Freud's writing is very different from the poet's attitude. His work also indicated, however, that where adult development has been faulty owing to a failure to leave behind infantile forms of sexual expression, wish-fulfilment and ego instinct, psychoanalysis could help that adult. It could guide him to an understanding of his own development, and suggest ways of overcoming personally those repressions of instinct and conflicts of inner self that have resulted from failure to mature properly. In other words, in connexion with the neuroses at least, Freud did not see his adults as tied irrevocably tightly to their infant and childhood sexual development.

This possibility of change and re-education in the adult is important, because Freud's work has in the past been used to reinforce the notion that individual development is over by the thirties and our habits and customs are irrevocably fixed by then. Such a notion is linked with the idea we have examined in an earlier chapter, that sexual tension and needs are maximum in youth and decline quickly towards middle age with absence of sex interest in old age.

In fact, as we have seen, middle age today brings the chances of further sexual development along with new ambitions and new patterns of social life. It also brings physical and emotional problems that require solving and settling but these, in themselves, are stimulants to change. The Swiss analyst C. G. Jung, who died only eight years ago, and who was a sympathetic follower of Freud until he founded his own analytical school, observed the significance of emotional and personality changes in the fourth decade of life. It has also been shown that middle-aged and older people can be retrained to different skills in different jobs where redundancy or ill-health has called for change of employment. The capacity to learn new skills has been found to depend less on the actual age in later years as on the educational level, mental attitude and the urge to work again.

There is no direct evidence from Freud's writings that he ever agreed with the notion of low sexual tension in middle age and an absence of sexual tension in old age. He treated

patients from a wide range of age groups and was just as
insistent on the sexuality of dreams and the conflict of ego
and libido in his older patients as in the younger ones. He
was scathing of contemporary physicians' recommenda-
tions that sexual abstinence was good for the individual's
health, and was one of the first doctors to stress the anxiety
and disturbance of sexual tension caused by the practice of
male withdrawal before emission in intercourse, known as
coitus interruptus.

In view of our earlier remarks about the sexual emancipation of women, towards which contemporary society is
rapidly moving via birth control, management of the menopause and better understanding of the female orgasm, the
attitude of Freud towards female sexuality is interesting.
While recognizing its importance for the health and integrity of the individual woman, it appears that he still saw the
female sexual role as essentially a passive one with gentle-
ness and warmth in the face of the male aggressiveness.
Also, far from preaching 'free love' and promiscuity as a
solution to sexual problems like repression and frustration,
his own life exemplified the possibility of monogamous
solutions.

Kinsey and Freud

The first copy of Kinsey's *Sexual Behaviour in the Human
Male* that I ever saw lay nestling among papers and magazines on the bench seat of a barber's waiting room. A curi-
ous resting place for this massive sex document of the
American male in his marital and extra-marital activities,
the barbershop was not really so inappropriate. After all,
it provided such intimate male articles as hair cream, razor
blades and rubber condoms for the customers. (I had a
similar experience in a way, when an article entitled 'Bald-

ness in the Elderly' which I published in a national journal turned up in the hairdressing and wig salon of a well-known Scottish hairdresser.)

As we have seen, Kinsey and his colleagues at Indiana University were not the first trail-blazers in search for the truth about sexual desires and activities. It is interesting to compare the impact which Freud's work and publications on psychoanalysis had on the First World War and post-war generations with that which Kinsey's work and publications had on the generations growing up after the Second World War. Both workers anticipated that the importance of their activities, and their published conclusions, would initially be obscured by the hostile reactions of a world still entrenched in strong sexual taboos. Both responded to this expected criticism in a similar way. They continued the work which they had initiated, and only considered constructive critical advice in pursuit of their goal – to increase sexual knowledge and understanding in and of man and woman. The reception of their work was unaffected by the fact that Kinsey was a zoologist with no medical degree, and Freud had a medical degree but welcomed lay pupils in his teachings of analytical methods.

Both men came to their important work in the sex field in an indirect manner. In Freud's case, he came to see the importance and influence of the sexual instinct while treating cases of neurosis as a practising medical man. In Kinsey's case, he came to see the need for expanding the knowledge on sexual behaviour when he became lecturer in charge of an official 'course in marriage' at the University of Indiana. Both lay and medical people often imagine that only the fully trained medical man can make reliable observations on the diseases and the health of the human body. History only partly confirms this view. Michelangelo showed us the path to true anatomy, Helmholtz demonstrated the retina with his mirror ophthalmoscope, Pasteur showed us the invisible miscrobes of disease, Sister Kenny showed us the proper therapy for 'infantile paralysis' patients and Pouseille showed us the path to measurement of blood pressure; yet none was a medical doctor.

In matters of sex, there have always been 'experts'. These may have been lay people who generalized on the basis of their own feelings and actions, not to mention their own education and upbringing, and whose knowledge of 'other practices' was minimal. Medical men, too, have been at a disadvantage since they see patients referred or coming because of sickness or difficulties. This gives them a biased and necessarily 'select' view of the patterns of sexual desires and sexual practices. It may not take account of the variations with age, education and religious upbringing which we have noted. Certainly it cannot encompass all those factors such as working life, childhood and adolescent experience, and leisure activities which determine the sexual *mores* of a given individual.

Born in 1856, Freud had a strict upbringing, yet his childhood conditioning did not prevent the flowering of his, at that time, unorthodox theories of sexuality in children. It was he who detected that the conscious and overt expressions of the sexual instinct exhibited in our civilization represent, like the visible portion of an iceberg, only a fraction of the whole. Below the surface lies a mass of unconscious, instinctive sexual drives implementing and supporting – and in some cases explaining – that which openly appears. Alfred Kinsey, born thirty-eight years after Freud, had a similarly orthodox upbringing, though the world of New Jersey was far different from the world of Freud's Vienna. He began as a scientific student in biology, and his early interest was in insect life, in particular the study of gall wasps. It was not till he became a lecturer in biology – having won his science doctorate – that the sexual iceberg began to command his interest. In this case, it was the statistical knowledge of sexual needs and sexual outlets in the Western world that lay mostly submerged under the water, with only a few facts surfacing now and then – like the studies of Exner and Pearl. Like Freud, Kinsey set about collecting histories of the sexual life – desires, attitudes, experiences, outlets – but this time on a scale which left all his predecessors far behind. The work which he began in 1937, and in which he was joined later by Wardell Pomeroy and Clyde Martin, was the most comprehensive objective search for factual knowledge in the sexual field that the scientific world had ever known. When their work first saw universal light of day with the publication by W. B. Saunders and Company of *Sexual Behaviour in the Human Male*, the volume ran to eight hundred pages of the most carefully collated facts, figures, explanations, ideas, and intensive statistical analysis of sex in the human male. Five years later, an equally large Volume on *Sexual Behaviour in the Human Female* revealed a similar assiduous collection of data on the thoughts, actions, deeds and desires of the other sex.

Many books and critiques of this outstanding work by Kinsey, who died in 1956, and by his associates at the Kinsey Institute, have been written, and much reappraisal of his information has gone on in the past two decades. One of the favourite criticisms was that Kinsey, Pomeroy and Martin gleaned their information as third parties and not as direct observers of the sexual behaviour which they noted down in their coded notebooks. Kinsey himself answered this criticism in several ways but agreed that the next project should be scientific observation of sexual practice, if possible in laboratory conditions. Nevertheless he had already observed sexual behaviour directly under different circumstances and through film and photograph. Another criticism was that implied in the best-selling novel, *The Chapman Report*, written by the distinguished author Irving

Wallace. The characters in his book bring out the point that human interpersonal relationships are more subtle than a mere record of sexual activities can suggest. The scientists are considered to have ignored the humanist element and not to have considered the emotion of love in the cold statistics of intercourse.

Among the facts and figures of Kinsey's original treatises, his study of sexual activity in the male showed its zenith in adolescence and a gradual decline into old age. He stressed what is now an accepted fact that the decline, though steady, does not show a fixed stopping-point in middle or old age. He considered that the gradual falling off in sexual activity was partly a question of 'capacity' (for the individual) and partly a question of 'psychological fatigue'. In the male, this latter expression included the emotional changes of middle age, the later climacteric, and the factors of familiarity, lack of 'new situations' and loss of novelty through repetition of approach. In his book he detailed the clues to sexual ageing which included, apart from the steady decline of frequency in sexual outlet, such factors as speed of erection, length of time that erection can be held, and the amount of mucus secreted in the outlet of the penis during the rising of the man's sexual tension. In the case of the female, his figures showed that the zenith of female sexual 'responsiveness' was in the late twenties but that the level of sexual tension increased in the thirties. Moreover, active sexual outlet in intercourse remains at a remarkably constant level into middle age in contrast to the steady decline in the male.

Kinsey's figures for people in the sixth, seventh and eighth decades of life were not really suitable for extensive statistical analysis because of the relatively small number of subjects in those older years who were interviewed. His information has, however, been ratified by other workers doing sex surveys.

Freud died in 1939 with the gratifying knowledge that his life's work on the basis of sexual instinct and sexual development had altered the entire fabric of society's attitudes to childhood and to adulthood. Kinsey's death nineteen years after, while he was still actively pursuing his goal of achieving the maximal knowledge of human sexual activity, left some unfulfilled projects. He could not know, but undoubtedly hoped, that these would be taken up by another observer of human nature who was scientifically and medically trained and eager for the truth.

A Prospect of Others

Field workers in the study of the ageing – doctors, sociologists, health visitors, psychiatrists and geriatricians – have all made personal and documented observations on sexual tension and sexual outlet in the aged. The president of the British Geriatrics Society, Lord Amulree, gave his own views on sex in the elderly in an important medical article in *The Practitioner* in the Spring of 1954. Dr Joan Malleson considered several aspects of sexual function in the older age group in her Penguin publication, *Change of Life*. The difficulty besetting professional men and women is the biased nature of the 'clinical material' which they usually have to study. This makes the determination of parameters for normal ageing and normal sexual needs and outlets in ageing more difficult to assess.

The value of preventive geriatric clinics lies not only in medico-social prophylaxis, but – because the attenders come voluntarily – the data obtained is from a more normal population and the information is more acceptable for statistical analysis and general application. Ideally then, a survey of sexual outlook and sexual function in the older age group – sixties to eighties – would cover a group of older people who can be considered as mentally and physically healthy in their status. Moreover, they would be in an outside community and not in an institutional atmosphere like that of a hospital or welfare old peoples' home. They should, like those attending the preventive clinic, enter the survey voluntarily, fully aware of the nature of the study and the reasons for its instigation. It is recognized that in any given group, some people will enter and then be reticent in answering more intimate questions – women are more likely to do this than men, at any age – and some allowance will have to be made for this.

The first study which approached these ideal conditions was made by Dr Gustave Newman and Dr Claude Nichols and published in the *Journal of the American Medical Association* in May 1960. They undertook a study of the sixty to eighty age-group in a group of geriatric subjects in a North Carolina community. Surveyed over a period of seven years this group showed the same characteristics (a gradual drop in sexual outlets and sexual tension with no sudden cessation of sexual activity and desire at a fixed chronological point) that we have noted from earlier studies. Further, the fact that, in any group of people, the range of sexual drive varies from very great down to very little, was shown to extend into the older age groups as well. In a personal unpublished survey of widowed or single people in institutional care, I noted a contrast between the lack of sexual interests, both towards self and towards the opposite sex, compared with the attitudes of married couples either in warden-supervised accommodation or in open houses, who still professed an interest in one another. The Newman and Nichols study stresses the importance of having a spouse with whom sexual activity is still possible, as an incentive to the continuation of sexual outlet.

I pointed out in an earlier chapter that ill-health or disablement at any age may result in a termination of sexual function in the form of coitus. Such termination may be recommended on medical grounds. Alternatively it may arise from the partners' mutual decision. As I said earlier, illness may be used as a convenient excuse. This study above confirms the pattern of illness and dysfunction physically reducing or stopping sexual outlet in the usual way, but also confirms that sexual tensions may still be active.

The anxiety and apprehension of older people who are aware of continuing sexual tensions and a desire for outlet – the guilt complex we have mentioned in an earlier chapter – was also observed by Dr Newman and Dr Nichols in their survey.

Perhaps the most important aspect of this survey is that it confirms that, in a healthy though ageing Western community, sexual activity can and does continue among married couples who so desire it, beyond the 'traditional' stopping-off age just after the menopause. Here again, the fact that an individual couple may vary from the conventional pattern does not make them 'normal' or 'abnormal', as if we must judge people against one standard.

In many communities, on both sides of the Atlantic, the medical training in sexual matters may be poor or, setting aside the teaching of the physiology of the sex organs and pregnancy, and some information on psychiatric abnormalities, virtually non-existent. It may represent a single lecture in the course on public health, or come up in the course of the training of medical jurisprudence for the medical undergraduate. This means that the family doctor, who, after all, is closest to his patients as people in a family unit, may have insufficient knowledge to give advice on sexual problems, or to take a proper sex history and know how to proceed on the basis of this information. While the patient may express himself or herself in vernacular terms, the doctor must learn and in turn teach the patient the proper terminology. This helps substantially to remove the atmosphere of emotional overlay that surrounds patient–doctor discussions on sexual problems. Today the knowledge of preventive aspects of conception is more widely available through family planning clinics and post-natal clinics. Also worthy of the doctor's interest and deeper research is an understanding of the varieties and techniques of the sex act. The need for 'experimental' patterns of sexual outlet in older or in disabled people, who still have sexual tensions, requires stressing. Studies like those of Newman and Nichols are an excellent guide for doctors who consider this aspect of daily living as important.

A Picture of Masters and Johnson

If Freud was the pace-setter on the understanding of sexual thought, and if Kinsey was the pace-setter on the collating of sexual facts, then their direct successors – this time as pace-setters in the visual understanding of the sexual act – must be Masters and Johnson. I have mentioned earlier that Kinsey answered some of his critics on the facts of the sexual act by suggesting the setting up of sex studies under physiology laboratory conditions. Thanks to Dr William H. Masters of Cleveland and St Louis, the unfulfilled plan for furthering sexual knowledge became a fruitful reality.

Qualifying first as a scientist (like the late Dr Kinsey) and later as a physician, Dr Masters went on to specialize in midwifery and in gynaecology and rose to the rank of consultant in this field of medicine. His decision to take up research into sexual function and activities is said to have been made at a much earlier age, but it was not until 1954 that he really began his laboratory project. One of the things which has amazed commentators on the Masters research programme is the fact that anyone or any couple would willingly volunteer to be directly observed in masturbation or in sexual intercourse, even if it was for 'the sake of science'. Part of the difficulty in accepting that normal healthy people would come and copulate in a laboratory – being filmed and having cardiograph and sphygmomano-meter readings made throughout the act – is that voyeurism is regarded in itself as a sexual deviation and is forbidden in religious and secular codes. (I have heard the comment that only deviationists or inverts would or could behave in such a fashion. Alternatively I have noted the naïve com-ment 'it could only happen in America'.)

Nevertheless, Dr Masters has been able to persuade heal-thy, normal (physically and sexually) people of all ages and all walks of life to visit his laboratory in strict privacy and take part in his research project. Accompanied by his research associate, Virginia Johnson, he began the pro-gramme of interviews and direct observations and record-ings in the research laboratory in the same year that Dr Alfred C. Kinsey died. Ten years later, the results of their work were published in the book *Human Sexual Response* and – as with Freud and Kinsey before – the world rocked on its axis at the intimate observations and detailed reve-lations, particularly on the long vexed question of female sexuality and female orgasm. Though their names have never become the sexual byword of the common man and the scientist, as did Kinsey's, they have been subjected to the same scorn, ridicule, harsh criticism and attempts to denigrate their work as Kinsey initially experienced. The same criticism of observing sex, and ignoring the humani-tarian and love aspects of sexuality in human relationships, has also been levelled at Masters and Johnson and their work at the St Louis laboratory. Needless to say, a novel which parallels their work has been written by another en-terprising author.

Several books and numerous articles and critiques – lay and medical – have been written about their work by people on both sides of the Atlantic. For details of their work, reference can be made to their own treatise or any of these books. From the aspects of the discussion on sex and the longer life which we have undertaken in this book, the most interesting observation was their confirmation that orgasm in older women was just as much possible as in younger women, even if, as would be expected, it was of lesser intensity. Their research continues and its findings will go on improving our understanding of the physiological sex mechanisms and outlets of human sexual tensions.

5 | The Changing Pattern

Inside Marriage

One of my favourite cartoons depicts an elderly gentleman, white-haired and obviously affluent, pressing his favours on a curvaceous young blonde as they sit over a night club dining table. The caption gives his words to her as, 'You see, my dear, my geriatrician doesn't understand me!' Apart from the play on the traditional phraseology of man on the make to girl on the take, the cartoon humorously strikes home two other points. It suggests in the first instance the truth of what we have clearly discovered in our discussions in this book – the older male still has sexual needs. Secondly, it suggests that older married people may find difficulties not only in their interpersonal relationships as a couple, but also in their communication with authoritative figures who can influence their sexual lives. On the latter point I have already stressed the lack of knowledge or training or both which may affect the physician's capacity as a sex counsellor, and the influence of establishment thinking on the usually conservative-minded doctors.

Throughout the preceding chapters I have generally assumed that the partners in our longer life will be 'life partners', that is, on the whole, that the sexual partners are wives and husbands rather than casual or paid sources of outlet. That this is a reasonable assumption until the sixth decade most people would agree. I have previously commented that life expectation in this decade has not really altered very much if at all. When you compare the sexes, however, you find that in the last ten years the expectation of life for women in the sixty-five to seventy-five age group has increased by fifteen per cent and for men not at all. This means that marriage terminating in widowhood is much commoner than that terminating in widowerhood. Thus the possibility of remarriage – and the continuation of a sex life within marriage – is potentially greater for women than for men. This makes our discussion on the menopause and post-menopausal years, in chapter 2, all that more significant. Incidentally, if traditional thinking considers the later years of marriage as 'sexless', it is even commoner to hear the expression 'platonic friendship' for remarriage in later life, implying the absence of sex needs for the couple.

The double bed versus single beds is a favourite theme of mine. The double bed is popularly understood as the expression of a sexually active married couple. If a married couple has separate beds it is assumed to be for one of three reasons. One or both of the partners is ill, or the partners are old (and by deduction impotent), or the partners are sexually incompatible. The idea propagated by Transatlantic movies that separate beds can be used successfully by 'happily married' couples was looked on askance by viewers on this side of the Atlantic. Innuendoes about catching cold on the way across, or the bedlinen on one of the beds never needing to be changed, ignored the comfort and hygiene of separate beds, particularly in hot climates. In the latter sense, the double bed is the Englishman's answer to his cold, damp and intemperate climate. Older people in this country are particularly resistant to dropping the double bed in favour of separate beds because of its implication of marriage difficulties. Thus I know of spouses sleeping in double beds where one partner is breathless with bronchitis or heart trouble, or restless with dementia, for example, who are sorely troubled at my suggestion of putting up a separate single bed for the ill spouse. Whether a

double bed does or does not help to maintain a better sexual relationship, and a happier married life for that matter,
is an arguable point in later married life. To some extent it
is coloured by the conventional view that the only 'proper'
place for sexual activity is in bed, at night, under the covers.
For an older couple, untroubled by children passing to and
fro or other such unwanted distractions, the warmth and
privacy of an evening by the fire (or should it be by the
central heating) is worth considering.

I recall attending a Furniture Exhibition in London some
years ago when a manufacturer was exhibiting what he
thought was the solution to the double versus separate
controversy. This consisted of twin beds set well apart,
which could, however, by means of an electrical button
switch at each bedside, be brought together as a double bed
when necessary. No prizes were offered in answer to the
question, what happens when one partner presses the
'together' button and the other presses the 'separator'
button at the same time?' Of course, this was necessarily a
rich man's answer and not for mass production but it did
highlight the point of view I have outlined.

Like most realistic observers, I am highly sceptical of
the statements made by fortunate couples celebrating their
golden and diamond wedding anniversaries that they have
never spoken a really cross word to each other or that they
have never had a violent argument or fallen out on any
occasion. Here the protective process of memory selectivity
recalls only the happy events; or the diminishing memory of later years, or even the glow of being in the limelight,
blurs the critical faculties of such long-married couples.
Newspapers and other mass media interviewers encourage
the couples in their self-deception as they feed the readers'
and listeners' own romantic marriage notions. No wonder
the song 'My old Duch(ess)' is perenially popular. The
truth is that long marriages like these demand a lot of

effort and mutual hard work to maintain them as the most desirable refuge for man and woman. Although virtually never mentioned by these older couples, sexual harmony at each decade of life and through each year of married life is a force for permanence within the bond.

As we have seen earlier, sexual difficulties are a feature in the lives of newly-wed and young married couples and this view is confirmed by sex counsellors and general marriage guidance counsellors. The resurgence of sex difficulties, as we have also noted, is liable to take place in later married life, because of the female menopause or, later, the male climacteric. There is no doubt that these difficulties tend to increase the likelihood of occasional or frequent infidelity, especially if the spouse adopts an attitude of *laissez faire* or indifference and, more so, if social opportunities allow. That a 'new, young' partner need not be the 'simple' answer, I have already stressed. Even if the new divorce laws make it somewhat cheaper and legally less difficult to break a marriage up at this age level, it would appear that many couples do not want to dissolve their marital status as the technically available solution of the moment to their sexual problems.

An alternative to cryptic infidelity that often reaches the Sunday press is open infidelity either by the introduction of a tacitly accepted 'third person' or the even more anti-biblical 'wife and husband swapping'. Presumably the equivalent in married couples of adolescent 'doing things for kicks', this exchanging of partners must make the maintenance of strong marital bonds all the harder for those who indulge in the practice.

The influence of living conditions on the stability of marriage is also important in the younger years. Overcrowding or poor sanitation or lack of household amenities, for example, may in turn influence the sexual outlets of the married couple. Conditions which deny a couple privacy for sexual activity, whether this is carried as far as inter-course or not, may create marriage difficulties. Similarly, persistently poor or awkward or overcrowded living conditions in later life can provoke the same sexual difficulties in marriage and neither spouse can even call upon the optimism (or ignorance, if you like) of youth to pursue a way out.

It would seem likely that parental influence might be less likely to provoke marital problems in later life. We have seen how the anti-sexual attitudes of mothers, not to mention mothers-in-law, can create early marriage difficulties. But a longer life means that middle-aged couples will often have very old parents to consider, and here again the responsibility and loyalty of either spouse to his or her parent(s) may put a strain on the marriage, including the sexual activity and outlet side. For example, I can recall talking to a middle-aged couple whose mother, in her eighties, had been admitted with pneumonia to the geriatric unit. They told me that she had lived with them for twenty-three of the twenty-six years of their married life and that this was the first time they had 'really had the house to themselves'. Both of them had sincere affection for the old lady but, as the wife further pointed her remarks, 'my husband and I have been closer these last few weeks than for many, many years'. Here, too, the post-war change from larger properties to small flats and houses enhances the family unit problems that arise down the years.

Not so very long ago, as the problems of an increasing elderly population were being considered by local authorities and their housing departments, the big trend was to the building of modern old peoples' welfare homes to house the pensioners whose slum property or oversized accommodation was unsatisfactory. Although most humane welfare authorities thought it was right to house husband and wife pensioners in the same hostel, there was rarely provision for true 'married rooms' in the homes.

Sex and the Longer Life

Matrons or superintendents of these homes, assuming a lack of sexual desire in these couples, were not unduly perturbed by the dissolution of the couple as partners. Since, as we have seen already, institutionalization does tend to diminish sexual desires, it is not surprising that the vocal complaints of such undeservingly treated couples were not more than a whisper in the course of time. Today the community care programme envisages more old people's bungalows or suitable flatlets which allow the maintenance of a couple's social – and if desired, sexual – integrity. The accommodation is lightly 'supervised' by enlightened wardens and not at all redolent of an institution. This is a welcome trend.

Outside Marriage

If, as we have suggested, the age difference between generally older husbands and generally younger wives combines with the decreased longevity of the husbands relative to their wives, then there is and will be a steady rise of widows in the community. To this may be added, if divorce becomes less difficult, more older men and women who have dissolved their matrimonial bonds. Still more, we can add the bachelors and spinsters of the longer life – those who have failed to reach marriage because of personality defects, peripatetic occupations, parental ties, career obligations or physical disabilities, for example. Most of these people will have some level of sexual tension throughout their lives and their sexual outlet will include coitus, masturbation, and erotic dreams although outside the 'legal' domicile of marriage. It seems invidious that such people should be subjected to an even stronger myth of sexlessness in older years than their married counterparts. I did point out in the previous chapter that lack of a marital partner does tend to reduce the coital sexual outlet in widowed or single older people. This does not mean that the other forms of sexual outlet are not used by both men and women. Unhappily, the attitude of society to these practices being what it is, more guilt and anxiety is engendered than even in the youthful non-coital outlet phase. This is unfair and oppressive and more likely to drive such parties to the venereal dangers of the casual contact or paid supplier.

I can almost hear a group of readers saying that there is an alternative in (what Freud is alleged to have called) sublimation. Releasing sexual tension through other non-sexual physical activity like charity work, club activities, part-time jobs, grandmotherly programmes, is the path of primroses specified. This is a reasonable solution for those with very low sexual tensions, but there are those who fail to 'sublimate' and for them erotic dreams or auto-erotic activities are a necessary outlet.

There are those, of course, whose outlet is that of the invert, whether this is male homosexuality or lesbianism. With few exceptions, society today still looks askance (if slightly more tolerantly towards women than towards men) at this form of outlet. There is no evidence that there is a sharp rise of inversion in older years – it is more likely that bisexual individuals cheated of a heterosexual partner by divorce or demise turn to the same sex for outlet.

Counsellors and Guiders

It is a traditional feature of the British way of life that whenever there is a social or socio-cultural problem of any magnitude within the national community, a group of people will come together at a local level to consider the problem and its possible solution. They will invariably set up a committee either before or after a conference initiated by the said group, and give themselves an explanatory title which they hope will rally support. Further publicity through press, radio (and nowadays television) is sought and branches are encouraged to grow throughout the country. As the committees grow in number, so the problem which they tackle is seen to be more widespread, more complex and greater in volume than first envisaged. This in turn leads the committee to become champions for a particular reform or new forms and to agitate as a group for pursuing these goals through Parliament to statutory acts.

The Old People's Welfare Committees and the Women's Royal Voluntary Service both arose in this way; similarly the National Marriage Guidance Councils have undergone their progressive growth after gestation. Originally a committee set up by the British Council for Social Hygiene, it took on its generic name in the year before the outbreak of the Second World War.

If we refer back to the religious codes of the three great monotheisms, Judaism, Christianity and Mohammedanism, and their three great tractates, the Old Testament, the New Testament and the Koran, we observe that 'marriage guidance' is an ancient practice in organized society. Moreover, the guidance is not just in sexual practice but also in social custom and in family tradition and in tribal etiquette.

Since, in all three religions, the male is the dominant power but the female is the key bond to the family, the marriage guidance rules lay particular stress on the feminine role. It is interesting therefore that the first post-war publication of the Marriage Guidance Council was called *How to treat a young wife.*

If we consider the question of marriage guidance purely from the sex counselling angle – and this appears to have been the approach of the original Council way back in 1938 – then we come across six popular ideas about sex counselling which are worth examining. In the first place, there is an idea that anyone can be a sex counsellor. Next, there is the suggestion that sex counselling is 'just commonsense'. Thirdly, there is the point of view that sex counselling is just another example of modern 'meddlesome do-gooding'. Next there is the idea that people inside or outside marriage should work out their 'own salvation' on sex matters. Then there is the suggestion that only doctors (who 'understand about sex') can give proper advice on sex. Lastly, there is the point of view that long-married people have nothing to learn or gain from sex counselling.

The idea that anyone can be a sex counsellor stems from the fact that sex, like eating food, is a universal pastime on which everyone has viewpoints. Given the juxtaposition of figure of authority to man in the street, or the know-all to the novice, then advice is very likely to be forthcoming, whether requested or not. Examples of these relationships are the minister of religion and the family doctor to their parishioners or their patients, by request, and parents and teachers to children and pupils, by arbitrary decision. Add to this the admonitions of mothers' circle and ladies' magazine on the one hand, and the counsel of masonic club and local pub on the other, and we can see why the uninitiated wonder why training is needed in such a simple matter as the giving of advice on sex.

The next suggestion, that sex counselling is 'just commonsense', is a direct corollary of the previous notion that anyone can be a sex counsellor. If you consider what we have already discussed on the questions of impotence and infertility alone, it should be obvious that commonsense is no substitute for factual assessment and applied knowledge. The danger of 'commonsense', as always, lies in applying popular conceptions (or as we have seen so far in the case of sex and ageing, popular misconceptions) as universal truths. If by commonsense we mean in addition the fruits of personal experience, here too we may run

125

aground if our personal experience is that of foul weather. Fortunately, as we have seen, pioneers like Kinsey and Freud early realized the value of collecting sexual information through factual histories so as to build up an enormous body of statistics, on which counsellors and guiders could draw when the practical moment of sex counselling came. Similarly, as a national body, the Marriage Guidance Councils have built up their own statistical records, which although concentrating on the causes of marital distress and break-up do include sex problems and sex difficulties. Further, Dr Masters is building up a pictorial library of the physiological mechanisms in sex function which can provide valid information to doctors as well as to non-medical counsellors.

The attitude that modern sex counselling is an example of 'meddlesome do-gooding' is not likely to be adopted either by those who have benefited from it or by those who are fully aware of the extent and limitations respectively in sex counselling. Couples where one partner feels that the other partner is 'entirely to blame' for sexual difficulties, are not likely to take kindly to counselling that makes them both look into their own behaviour and feelings. Similarly an aggrieved spouse who is sure that the counsellor will encourage her to take one line of action, may be surprised at the impartial approach to the situation which is adopted. The 'mind your own business' attitude is very familiar to the man from the 'Cruelty' called in by neighbours when parents are mistreating their offspring. The same attitude may be adopted when one married person seeks help and then asks the spouse to attend the counsellor, at the latter's request, only to receive the rejoinder that he or she is not interested in meddlesome do-gooding.

An extension of this attitude may involve a fear that the information supplied will affect the moral security of the individual or his or her spouse, or undermine the dominant position of the male partner. There is no doubt that some of the opposition to Family Planning clinics arose from such misgivings on the sexual score in the marriage symphony, on the part of secular and religious groups as well as individuals.

Doctors as professional counsellors in many matters other than sex are also aware of the reverse approach – that is, the seekers of advice affirm that they are delighted with the offer of 'helpful advisement'; they then proceed to demonstrate that covertly or openly they wish to finesse the doctor into playing the patient's cards for him. Thus the question, 'what do you think we should do, doctor' becomes rhetorical to the patient's preplanned answer. Doctors usually recognize when they are being manipulated and, with training, turn it to good use in their assessment of patients and situations from the emotional and medical aspects. The untrained 'commonsense counsellor' quickly falls into the trap and wonders why he finds his hands tied and his mind in a whirl.

The next idea, that people inside or outside marriage should work out their own sexual salvation, has, on the face of it, much to commend it. Maturation of the partners in a marriage calls for mutual consideration, mutual adjustment and bilateral determination to make it reasonably happy and reasonably successful. The 'running home to mother' approach of either partner in early married life may be allowable once and once only, but from then on working it out together should replace the in-law as weapon tack. We have noted, however, that sexual difficulties may spring from sexual ignorance. Even 'with it' 'on the pill' wives may be remarkably uninstructed and raw on anatomy, physiology, technique and psychology of sexual life and equally so their 'with it' 'been around' husbands: so too for boyfriends and girlfriends. To ask such people to struggle on unaided into a bigger mess is most unfair, if not unrealistic. Moreover, as we have discovered, ignorance of sexual changes in later life and the possibility of overcoming them can lead to difficulties at a point in the marriage when the need for sex counselling – at least in the practical sense – might be unexpected.

The idea that only doctors can give proper advice on sex matters has some historical backing. In modern times, at least, if you include doctors of philosophy and doctors of biology as well as doctors of science – the names of Marie Stopes, Isadore Rubin and Kenneth Walker are conjured up to mind as examples – then sex counselling by doctors has been important and progressive and socially effective. The deficiencies of training in sex matters in many medical schools on both sides of the Atlantic does not preclude a biology or science or medical degree as a valuable fundament to the fabric of sexual knowledge and, in turn, to sex counselling. The Marriage Guidance Councils have found, however, that a multidisciplinary approach to marriage and sex problems has greater sociological and ethical value as well as being practical. Thus doctors and clergymen, solicitors and headmasters, social workers and nurses, may all act in a consultative capacity in a given problem or number of problems. In fact, the counsellors trained in marriage guidance by the council come from no specific occupational group and need not have a degree in medicine, science or biology. It is a question of personality, attitude and stability combined with sufficient education, rather than the 'initials' after one's name.

Lastly, there is the attitude that long-married people have nothing to gain from sex counselling. I hope I have dwelt sufficiently in the earlier chapters on the sexual problems and possible therapies in the older person, to make it clear that sex counselling is valuable to married people at any age. There is no reason either why older widowed or single people should not also benefit from sex counselling in the light of modern attitudes to sexual outlet and tensions. It is true that older people are less inclined to come forward for fear of being mocked or ridiculed or misunderstood. They may also not take kindly to advice or counsel from a 'young whippersnapper' or 'young know-all'. The need for kindness, tact, sympathy and a positive optimism in sex counselling for older people is all the more important on that account. It is no good having a welfare state which sees generously to the material needs of its members but puts up a barrier to caring for their spiritual and psycho-sexual needs.

Inside the Geriatrician

The changing pattern in our attitude to older people is partly reflected in the growth of gerontology and of geriatrics. The former involves studying the ageing processes in animals and in man and trying to understand what is involved both at the level of tissues and cells, and at the level of chemical and biochemical changes within the cells. If this appears a little like the alchemists' search for the 'elixir of life' during the Dark and Middle Ages, the difference lies in the unhurried approach, the use of scientific method and the recognition that at the present time, and in the foreseeable future, there is still a finite limit to human life round about the hundred and tenth year.

Geriatrics is a relatively new branch of general medicine which has developed over the past two decades. It involves the study of diseases and disabilities in the older members of the population. The physician trained in this speciality, and often called a geriatrician, learns the art and skill of diagnosis and treatment of sickness and disablement in the over-sixties. He undertakes such therapy in his own special unit, called a geriatric unit, in the general hospital. In my previous book, *Later Life – Geriatrics Today and Tomorrow*, I outlined the aims of contemporary geriatrics and of the practising geriatricians both at home and in hospital. In a nutshell, this involves trying to maintain older people during the treatment of illness or disabilities which confine them to bed or prevent them moving about their normal daily activities. If admission to hospital is required, the geriatric unit undertakes a programme of positive rehabilitation on a 'progressive patient care' basis.

In the course of that book, I explained what an uphill struggle it has been, and often still is, to make old age a popular cause and the active optimistic treatment of illness in old age a viable activity. The geriatrician has to be constantly on guard against the 'what does it matter at that age' outlook and 'the money would be better spent on younger people' attitude. The more that general medicine advances in such important and dramatic fields as organ transplantation, artificial kidney therapy and radioactive beam treatments, for example, the harder the geriatrician has to fight for the right of simple unspectacular needs of geriatric unit wards, like adequate nursing staff and modern beds and bathrooms.

Geriatrics differs from general medicine in several ways. The most important of these is the influence which social (and economic) circumstances have on the patient's illness and the need for his or her admission to hospital. Thus geriatric problems are invariably medico-social problems and require a team – doctors, nurses, medico-social workers, health visitors and others – to solve the patient's illness and difficulties in the best and most constructive way. Sexual problems based on physical disease processes like, for example, arteriosclerotic dementia or lack of pituitary hormone, are tackled by the geriatrician as part of the general approach to the disease process. No special training in the sex needs and sex problems of older people is normally given, although once again medical knowledge plus experience plus pragmatism may be used to give advice and answer appropriate questions.

In the ordinary way, geriatricians are concerned with diseases or disturbances that have already occurred. The preventive aspect is usually the province of public health departments of local authorities. Since the establishment of the Rutherglen Preventive Geriatric Clinic in 1952 in Glasgow, the idea of preventive geriatrics has steadily grown. The introduction of questionnaires, which include requests for help or discussion of sexual needs and sexual outlets, has begun in several clinics but its importance is still rated relatively low. The knowledge of normal ageing processes is still limited. Further, the difficulties of ensuring adequate diagnosis and treatment of disease in older people, not to mention the preventive aspect, are still to be overcome. It is hardly surprising then that consideration of sexual needs or sexual problems in the longer life is not a major item in the geriatrician's world. Nevertheless, just as the geriatrician has had to take decisions on who will benefit from treatment of physical disease or rehabilitation therapy of disabilities, in time he is likely to be called upon to decide on the advisability of female sex hormone and male sex hormone treatment, in appropriate cases. Moreover, if sex training is included for those geriatricians involved in preventive geriatric work, this will provide an important 'advice bureau' for those who, in the ordinary way, might be wary of attending 'sex advice clinics' boldly so named.

It might be thought, on the other hand, that since sex is a psycho-physical function, the proper person to act as guide and instructor should be the doctor trained in psychological medicine, namely the psychiatrist. Certainly men and women who are referred by their family doctors under the Health Service to a psychiatrist, or who seek private consultation with a psychiatrist, often have sexual disturbances or difficulties as the primary presenting symptom. In that sense, the doctor in psychological medicine is likely to be asked for help in apparent or real cases of sexual abnormality. The problem of what is and what is not a sexual abnormality or aberration (perversion is the favoured expression) is a function of the time, place and society in which the person lives, or the partner with whom the man or woman cohabits. I have already stressed the point that masturbation, which was regarded as a sexual aberration a century ago, is now well understood to be a normal sexual outlet.

If a patient's sexual activities disturb his or her partner, however, not so much because they usually practise patterns that are foreign to the complainant but because they are indulging in new unacceptable habits, a psychiatric opinion may be called for. The difficulties over impotence and frigidity may also cause the partner or partners to seek psychiatric help and this approach may reveal evidence of illness such as psychoneurosis requiring psychotherapy and drug treatment. Men, in particular, with low sexual tension and low levels of output, may be found to have a neurosis that may or may not be amenable to treatment. We have commented earlier that patients with mental illness may suffer from altered libido, or ascribe their depressed state to the effects of 'sexual excess' or 'sinful sex' which is, to the mentally healthy observer, far from the truth. In all these cases, psychiatric help is invaluable. In the case of the anti-social or psychopathic individual, where action and reaction in the social sphere is often violent or cruel, the sexual relationship at any stage will be unstable and liable to show evidence of aggression. Psychotherapy may or may not be very successful but the interested psychiatrist may be willing to try and help in any case.

One of the features of ageing is the narrowing effect on personality and dislike of change. We have seen how a change in sexual pattern, on the other hand, can be helpful in maintaining or improving sexual relations in the longer life. To balance these opposing patterns, education and early relearning activities in connexion with sexual practice are necessary for more successful sexual adjustments in older couples. In such re-education, the non-medical psychologist must also have an important role, integrated with the help of psychiatrist, geriatrician and family doctor. Such a sex education council is partly inherent in marriage guidance councils but its work should be more concentrated on the 'neglected' older years.

Health versus Sex

The most obvious argument against sexual practice like coitus in later years is the rising incidence of physical and mental disease in people as they grow older. Mental ill-health in the over-sixties, such as anxiety states, neuroses, depression or paranoia for example, have been variously estimated to affect from ten per cent to forty per cent of the population at risk. Physical illness like heart disease, chest disease and brain disease is also commoner in a greater percentage of the over-sixties than in the first four decades of life. The old primitive belief – still a feature of some religions – that emission of semen for men or regular coital activity for both sexes is 'weakening' or 'life-shortening' has no substance in scientific fact. It has been a useful 'idea' for those who think that abstinence is a more spiritual act than physical sexual outlet. It has been an even more useful 'threat' of parents, teachers and religious instructors to the pubescent and adult young, and of the establishment towards the lower social classes. It is interesting how all these groups which are and have been anti-sex at one time or another are quite sure that physical activity of the nongenital muscles – sports and athletic pursuits – are health-giving to mind and body at all ages. Perhaps the fact that sexual activity is an indoor 'sport' while most others are outdoor in the fresh-air and sunshine, plus the notion that sex is personal to one or two people while outdoor sport is gregarious and competitive, adds to the attitude that health and sexual activity are somehow incompatible. This is not to deny that muscular sports do improve health and help guard against several illnesses, as the Framingham study in the United States has shown. But if regular activity of the limb muscles maintains tone and improves strength and efficiency, it must surely be a corollary that regular sexual activity maintains genital muscle tone and improves sexual performance and sexual outlet. Both the Kinsey and New-man–Nichols surveys have shown clearly that the greater the frequency of sexual outlet, particularly coitus, main-tained from early marriage days, the more likely that coitus will have a higher frequency in later life. Moreover, the usual tapering off of activity, at a gradual rate, will be slower in those couples who have been most active sexually in their earlier married life.

I have already touched on the problem that ill-health may present in partners who wish to continue their conjugal activities as well as their general marital partnership. In the acute phase of mental or physical illness, sexual tension is generally low or absent (except in some abnormal sexual responses as in dementia) and no warning from doctors is required to ensure abstention. It is in the post-acute phase of the illness, or in the interim phase between acute attacks, or in the long-term slight or moderate disability phase, that difficulties can and do arise. The doctor is aware that sexual tension that is not relieved by sexual outlet can produce general body tension, anxiety and frustration, irritability and restlessness. Although the evidence is not conclusive in every case, it is generally accepted that such emotional stress aggravates blood vessel illness, such as high blood pressure, angina and coronary artery disease, not to mention stomach ulcers and colitis.

On the other hand, doctors are aware that normal marital coitus, involving initial love-play, excitement and the orgasmic phases, calls for a substantial output of physical energy. Also the physical tension stimulates the adrenal glands and sympathetic and parasympathetic nerves, making the systolic blood pressure rise several points, the pulse and heart rate increase quite markedly, the breathing rate increase and the skin flush over. In the case of people suffering from chest disease, like chronic bronchitis, the effort of full coitus may provoke excessive and uncomfortable breathlessness. Or in the case of people who have chest pain (angina) on effort, coitus may provoke an anginal attack. It is because of this that doctors may reply strongly in the negative if casually asked about resumption of sexual relations after pneumonia or a heart attack, for example. More careful assessment of the patient's usual sexual needs and outlet may show that a short period of abstinence could be followed by a return to occasional coitus, if necessary omitting the love-play. Or the physician may recommend coitus in a more relaxing position – say, side-to-side or from the rear – provided both partners have no untoward objection to this. Since the stimulation of the sympathetic nerves in the case of the male – and in middle age it is more likely to be the male that has arterial disease – lasts only a short time, the rise in heart rate and blood pressure is not likely to be prolonged.

Again, as I have explained before, the illness may be chosen as the 'sexual breaking-off point for the partner'. This is likely not only in the previous unhappy sexual set-up but where either or both partners are genuinely frightened of recurrence of chest, heart, ulcer or colon trouble if sexual relations are actively renewed. Obviously there can be no hard and fast rules about resuming coitus after an illness or in the long-term disablement phase. If sexual tensions do appear they will need to be dealt with accordingly. The patient's doctor may prescribe tranquillizers or barbiturates to help suppress libido and the need for outlet, if asked to do so or if he thinks it necessary. Alternatively, he may suggest cautious 'trial and error' if both partners are keen to enjoy sex with each other. If nothing is said and the patient assumes coitus is 'out', he may still (or she may still) find outlet in masturbation, wet dreams or physical contact so that excitation still occurs, even if the doctor is not 'aware' of it.

A major psychological barrier in sexual activity may be the presence of physical disability, physical disfigurement and altered physiological functions, in either or both partners. For example, a patient suffering from joint disease in the hips or back may be too disabled to enjoy sexual intercourse in the popular position of man over woman with the woman's legs extended. Psychologically he or she may dislike an alternative posture and position which, though technically satisfactory, makes him or her feel guilty of somehow 'letting the partner down'. In the case of physical disfigurement, the result of external trauma like burns or external physical disease like warts or growths may be to upset the partner by embarrassment or even revulsion. This may be overcome by gradual adjustment to the altered appearance over a period of months and the slow but steady loss of embarrassment. Alternatively it may permanently split the partners and be a cause for separation in married couples.

In the rarer cases of altered physiology, such as the replacement of rectal excretion of faeces by an abdominal exit called colostomy, the problem may be one of embarrassment both on the patient's part – worry about possible odour and 'accidents' – and the partner's part. This may result in temporary or permanent psychologically-based impotence in the male and frigidity in the female. Again, after some months, both patient and partner may become adjusted to the presence of a colostomy and gradually resume sexual relations. Alternatively, the partner's upset at the bowel opening in the abdominal wall may never be completely overcome, and sexual relations are either minimal or absent from then on.

Mild physical disease or physical disability may also prove a barrier to sexual relations where there is an associated mental disturbance such as anxiety neurosis or in the personality disintegration of the dementias or in the true psychoses such as melancholia and schizophrenia. Here, resumption of coital activity is likely to be difficult, and sometimes impossible.

Tempo Andante, Con Variazioni

When I first came to Lancashire, I had been warned to expect a grimy exterior and a warm interior. The former applied to the buildings and factories and the latter to the people who worked in them. What I was not cautioned about was the dry straight-faced sense of humour among Lancastrians, particularly among the older generations. On one occasion I was asked to see a man living in a slum property whose family doctor told me that the patient was bronchitic and required early hospitalization for treatment of his chest and under-nutrition. When I visited the grimy terraced cottage, I found him in a double bed with an equally chesty and under-nourished looking old lady. I examined the man and casually, by way of conversation, I smiled at the old lady and said to the man, 'And that'll be your missus, then?' The old gentleman shook his head, coughed once and said, 'Nay, doctor, we're just good friends.' Such is the leg-pulling of many a spouse in the old people of Lancashire.

I recall this story whenever people question the idea that marriage in the later years is anything more than a monotonous habit or a dull companionship, and that the idea of sexuality in older people is either untrue or socially very unlikely. It is admitted that patches of any marriage must be monotonous or dull and that the sexual spark may be dampened or less easily ignited at various times. To condemn older people to dullness or asexuality just because of society's expectations or lack of them is unfair and unwarranted, as I hope I have made clear in the preceding chapters.

There are a number of difficulties which, we have seen, will tend to interfere with sexuality in later married life. We have mentioned the hormonal changes, earlier in women, later in men, and how these may possibly be overcome. Also, we have mentioned the effects of illness, both physical and mental, and of disabilities within the marriage framework, not forgetting poor accommodation and strained economic or social circumstances. The contrast between the declining economic power of the over-sixties – the first impoverished leisure generation as they have been called – and the rising economic power of the adolescent generations lies not only in material welfare but in sexual welfare as well. Again, we have considered how the effects of illness on sexual relations can be influenced or overcome in appropriate cases.

There are other disadvantages under which many members of the present older generation labour. For many of them, formal education may have ceased at thirteen and sexual education has often been no more than illicit books, blue jokes and some hasty advice from parents or friends just prior to marriage. The women will have been brought up with a stricter morality, and the effects of aggressive male sexuality may have been permanently to impair their desire for coitus. Marriage itself will have been an 'education' but not necessarily of the most helpful, informative or edifying type. Despite menstruation and childbirth, there is a remarkable lack of knowledge of female and male anatomy and physiology among women, and equally so among men. The prudery of previous generations with regard to woman's underwear, and to the naked body, is often uninfluenced by long years of marriage.

For example, a man aged sixty-nine, a retired miner, developed a cancer of his left lung. This proved after investigation to be inoperable and he was sent back home for his wife, who was sixty-five, to take care of him. The miner and his wife had five children, all grown up and married, who lived fairly near and helped the miner's wife in various ways. After eight months, he developed a spread of the cancer to his brain and became paralysed on the left side. He became completely bedfast and at times was incontinent. His wife refused the help of the district nurse because, she said, she could do 'all the necessary' and her husband did not like the idea of a female, even if she was a trained nurse, attending to him. Eventually the burden of terminal care did become too much for her, and the local geriatrician was requested to provide a 'terminal care' bed. On his assessment visit, he commented how well the wife had looked after the miner. She acknowledged this and remarked, 'I didn't think I could manage it. He and I have always been shy about each other, and I have seen more of him in the past few weeks than in all our married life.'

By contrast, the younger generation regard nudity in sex relations as natural. The success of naturist groups shows that the hidden fear of clothed people, that nakedness may encourage continuous sexual stimulation in a mixed community, is only a function of their misguided logic that clothes prevent promiscuity.

Another anti-sex factor influencing the older generation was the effects of venereal disease. This was more likely to be a point influencing them against casual sexual contacts or promiscuous extra-marital behaviour. The verbal weapons of the anti-sex establishment groups included the threat of general paralysis of the insane, ulceration, and sick offspring, all from the effects of a syphilitic infection. The dangers of gonorrhoea, producing damage to the tubes and infertility in women, urethritis in men, and blindness in the newborn, were also stressed. These terrors were used to intimidate not only those who engaged in extra-marital sex but also those who might otherwise enjoy regular cohabitation in the marriage bed. If the married male partner was a 'traveller' of the commercial or military or marine type, the link was clearly more dismaying. The coming of penicillin and the antibiotics has certainly lowered the venereal disease rates for syphilis and gonorrhoea (but not for non-specific urethritis) and has made the traditional bogy of these illnesses much less, if not little, for the sons and daughters of today.

This brings us on to the sexual morality of the older generation. We have already touched on the influence of orthodox religion on the view of sex in marriage. This, we have seen, came down strongly to stress the procreative side of sex rather than sex as a pleasurable expression of affection between a man and his wife. Further, religious orthodoxy views virginity in the prospective bride as highly important, and premarital sex, even among the affianced, as sinful. Christian theologies follow the earlier Judaic code in underlining the requirement that the married man and his wife take part in sexual intercourse with one another only when both agree to this. This recognizes that conception may not be the main goal of the act for the individual couple but is still the spiritual objective from the religious standpoint. Infertile couples are not therefore denied a sex life at least while either partner is in the fruitful years. In viewing sex as a means to a procreative end, it would be logical for orthodox religious people to give up sexual activity as soon as the wife reaches her menopause. This ignores the continuation of sexual tensions and sexual needs by either or both partners and, on that basis alone, it is hardly surprising that the secular view of sex as physical love with the incidental benefit of children, where desired, tends to prevail.

The above is not an argument against religious doctrine as such. Religious belief has always contained valuable moral notions as well as notions which do not fit into contemporary understanding of physical and mental human activities. If religion accepts the idea of sex which is secularly practised as above, its most effective standpoint still lies in insisting that the marriage framework is the best structure within which sexual expression can blossom for mutual benefit. That this idea is acceptable even to the radical youth of today is expressed in the high under-twenty marriage rate.

It may be a criticism of this book that there is 'too much stress on sex in marriage' whatever the age of the couple. Marriage is more than just physical intimacy and sexual exploration, of course. The point of concentrating on Sex in the Longer Life in this book is to help remove the myths and misunderstandings which I have outlined, and let sexual function be a smoother and more naturally progressive side of marriage than heretofore. It is also to stress the need for better sex education in older people, both medical and non-medical, so that sex counselling can be more effective and helpful.

At the same time, we must recognize that many marriages, both before and after the menopause, function apparently successfully with no sexual contact of the partners or with minimum sexual outlet in coitus. Even so, for the large majority of married couples, sex is important in maintaining a stable relationship and a satisfactory inter-personal bond.

Two other factors are of interest and I would like to mention these. Nearly twenty years ago, Hans Selye, a brilliant physiologist, was working on the problem of how the human body reacted to stress and stressful situations. There were many ideas at the time. These included the importance of the sympathetic nervous system (which, we have seen, has also an important function in sexual physiology) as a 'fight or flight' mechanism. The nerves gave an alarm reaction which toned up muscles, increased the heart rate and the blood pressure and the breathing rate and made the person 'ready for anything'. A second important system was the humoral one in which adrenaline and noradrenaline were released by the adrenal glands, lying above each kidney, and these hormones also produced an alarm reaction with hair standing up and sweat pouring out. A third theory gave pride of place to the pituitary gland in the brain. This small gland was stimulated by visual signs through the eye nerves, or auditory signs through the ear nerves, or tactile signs through the skin nerves, and set off chemical messenger hormones to the other (adrenal, thyroid) hormone glands. The pituitary also triggered off the sympathetic nerves.

The theory of Hans Selye, known as the General Adaptation Syndrome, showed how the human being reacted to stress by linking all three systems into the hypothalamic – pituitary – adrenal axis. This produced not just adrenaline and noradrenaline for 'fight or flight' but, just as important, it produced cortisol from the adrenal cortex. It is cortisol and its homeostatic analogues that counteract shock and strain, in the stress situation.

It is often thought that older people's stress axes must be deficient because of their often more serious response to illness and slower recovery. If this were true, then the sexual response might also be expected to be less since the same axis is tied up with sexual physiology. In fact, recent research by a geriatrician based on hormonal measurements before and after stimulation of the axis, has shown the integrity of this axial anti-stress mechanism until the ninth decade. So it is not surprising, after all, that sexual function can be effective so late in the human life.

The other interesting factor is the idea, occasionally expressed, that a spouse can become 'allergic' to the partner just as some human beings become allergic to cats or dogs with whom they live. Now allergy is usually based on the development in the blood of protein factors, called antibodies. These clash with the activating protein antigens and produce a hypersensitivity reaction of rashes, swelling of tissue, weakness and collapse. Hay fever is an example of allergy to grass antigens, which is milder than the reaction just described. It so happens that the seminal fluid of man contains protein and, in theory, a wife who developed antibodies to the seminal fluid might show allergic features on intercourse in the absence of a condom. At the time of writing only one such case has been substantiated in literature. This is a remarkable tribute to nature, which seems to have ensured that even after many years of cohabitation in marriage, that sort of allergy is extremely rare. Psychological 'allergy' is quite a different matter and would call for a psychiatric assessment and help. It can be important, as we have seen, in some cases of male impotence towards the wife.

Franz Schubert, who never came to enjoy the longer life, composed a delightful quartet in D minor, in whose second movement the tempo is marked 'andante, con variazioni'. I can think of no better instruction for marital maintenance of sexual interest and pleasure than Schubert's musical advice: a steady pace, with variations on the theme.